The Diabetic Nutribullet Recipe Guide:

100+NutriBullet Diabetes Blasting Ultra Low Carb Delicious and Health Optimizing Nutritious Juice and Smoothie Recipes

Sione Michelson

Disclaimer

Preview (Protein Pack)

- 3 cups of spinach
- 1/2 cup of strawberries
- 2 Tbsp. Peanut Butter
- A small piece of ginger
- 1/2 cup of blueberries
- 1 cucumber

Health Benefits:

One cup of spinach has almost 20% of the RDA of dietary fiber, which helps in digestion, prevents constipation, maintains low blood sugar, and curbs overeating. Studies have also shown that the consumption of spinach may also reduce the risk of prostate cancer. I try to put spinach in all my juices because it has so many great health benefits.

Preview (Mint Explosion)

- 1 avocado
- 1 handful of mint
- 1 cup spinach
- 1 cup parsley
- 1/2 cup of strawberries

Health Benefit: Avocados are high in beta-sit sterol, a compound that has been shown to lower cholesterol levels. I love to add avocados to most of my juices because they are a great source of protein which is great for muscle recovery after an intense workout.

Get All My Books to Help in Mastering your Life Today

JUICING: THE ULTIMATE BEGINNERS GUIDE FOR JUICING WITH THE NINJA BLENDER & NUTRIBULLET (OVER 60 RECIPES NEW!!!!)) (Juicing, Juicing for Weight Loss, Books, Recipes, ... for Weight Loss, Women's Health Diet)

Paleo Diet:: Learn How to Lose Weight and Feel Amazing in just 5 Short Weeks. The Quickest way to Fit into that Swimsuit for Summer! (Paleo Made Easy) (Paleo ... Diet, Slow Cooker, Recipes, Diet Recipes)

Paleo Diet: Why The Paleo Diet is better for you than the Low Fat High Carb Diet & the Paleo Recipes that will help Save Your Life! (Paleo Cookbook, Weight-Loss, ... Diet, Slow Cooker, Recipes, Diet Recipes)

Paleo Diet: 7 Days To Better Health: Cure Your Acid Reflux, Heartburn, Start losing Weight, Lower Blood Pressure and Cholesterol All in a Week through ... Diet, Slow Cooker, Recipes, Diet Recipes)

Juicing: The Ultimate 7 Day Juicing Cleanse for Weight-loss Guide: Over 60 Delicious Juicing Recipes made with the Nutribullet and Ninja. Increase Metabolism ... Weight Loss, Women's Health Diet Book 1)

Juicing: The Ultimate 7 Day Juice Challenge: (60+recipes!!) To help Lower your Blood Pressure, Cholesterol, Acid Reflux and Start Losing Weight all with ... Weight Loss, Women's Health Diet Book 1)

The Low Carb Nutribullet & Ninja Recipe Book: 10 day juice cleanse: 100+ Health Sustaining Low Carb and Delicious and Nutritious Juice and Smoothie Recipes ... for Weight Loss, Women's Health Diet)

Juicing: The Only Juicing for Health Guide You Will Ever Need:100 + Juicing and Smoothie Recipes for Weight Loss, Lower Blood Pressure, Reduce Acid Reflux ... for Weight Loss, Women's Health Diet)

Juicing for Health: The Ultimate Juicing Guide for Optimal Health: Start Feeling Better your Very First Day: 100+ Easy To Follow Nutribullet & Ninja Recipes. ... for Weight Loss, Women's Health Diet)

Juicing for Fat Loss: The Ultimate Juicing Guide for Fat Loss: A complete 10 Day Juicing Guide that is Sure to Help You Lose Fat and Keep it off for Good!

Juicing For Beginners: The Easiest Juicing Guide Ever Made, 100+ Delicious Juicing and Smoothie Recipes for Optimal Health, Lower your Blood Pressure & ... for Weight Loss, Women's Health Diet)

Juicing: Juicing for Vitality: 7 Days to a Better Life, Drastically Improve your Energy, Lose Weight, Improve Sex Drive, Improve Skin Complexion and Much ... for Weight Loss, Women's Health Diet)

Juicing: Juicing for Weight Loss: 5 Days to Better Health, Easy to Follow Steps and Recipes: Lose Weight & Improve Your Health all by Taking Action Today! ... for Weight Loss, Women's Health Diet)

Table of Contents

Book link/Social media

Since I've dedicated my life to personal growth, health and life mastery, I felt I must add this other book that deals with overcoming social anxiety, shyness and low self-esteem. Did you know that 1 in 3 people deal with these issues? Here are some great lessons in this E-book that help with that.

Shyness

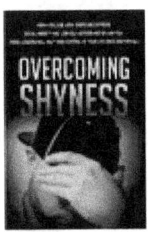

Follow me on Facebook and Twitter to see what other books are in the works!

Facebook: Sione's Facebook

Twitter: Sione's Twitter

Introduction

First of all I want to thank you for purchasing my book but you should really be thanking yourself for taking the initiative towards good health. Today begins the first day of the rest of your life. The rest of your life can be the best of your life if you just stay consistent with your diet and exercise. The best way to start to do this is through the great benefits of juicing daily.

Juicing for diabetics can be extremely helpful in controlling blood glucose levels. Fresh vegetable juice is loaded with antioxidants, phytochemicals, It is beneficial for normalizing blood sugar, plus fresh vegetable juice can be a key ingredient in a healthy weight loss program. You will begin to notice positive changes such as better moods and clearer skin as you start to and continue to eliminate harmful toxins from your body. You will also be lowering you cholesterol & blood pressure all the while losing weight at the same time and these delicious juicing & smoothies will help you do just that. I've have even add a !!!!BONUS 40 + PALEO & SLOW COOKER RECIPES!!! This book has it all in one spot! Your one-stop-shop towards health. It's time to enjoy the rest of your life!

Preparation for all recipes

Get yourself a really good blender. I like to use the Ninja because it blends my food up really nice. You may need to cut fruit and veggies in halves or quarters, it's probably wise to pre-package all your cut up fruit, put them in individual zip lock bags and store them in the freezer. This will help save you lots of time and hassle instead of having to do this every day, plus cutting up your fruit into smaller pieces will keep the food from jamming up the blender. For the most part the Ninja will blend up lots of whole fruits and veggies; it also has no problem blending up ice! I like to add between a ¼ to a 1/2 cup of ice to each juice because this makes a refreshing smoothie. If your juice ends up being too bitter try adding some bananas, this helps reduce the bitterness nicely!

Juice Power

The Simplicity recipe is a quick and easy juice I prepare for them mornings when I wake up late and have to be to work.

- 2 carrots
- 1 apple
- 1/2 cucumber

Health benefits:

Skin benefit: Carrots contain vitamin A and other antioxidants, which helps prevent wrinkling, skin dryness, skin blemishes and uneven skin tone.

Fruit Paradise

I use this recipe when I want to make sure I got all the nutrients I need for the day.

- 2 apples
- 2 oranges, peeled
- 2-4 stalks of celery
- 1/2 cup of parsley
- 1 cucumber
- 1 lemon, unpeeled
- 1 small piece of ginger

Health Benefits:

Celery can help you lose weight because it makes you feel full without consuming many calories. Celery will also help you get your fluid needs as it is comprised of over 90% water. Having enough water in your body helps your workouts last longer. When you are properly hydrated it takes longer for muscle fatigue to set in.

Antioxidant Machine

- 3 carrots
- 1 large beet
- 2-4 stalks of celery
- A handful of parsley
- 1 lemon, unpeeled
- 1-2 cloves garlic

Health Benefit: Parsley's powerful oils can be an excellent health benefit because it is loaded with helpful antioxidants that help prevent cell damage which is a key in fighting cancer.

Kale Beginner

- 4-7 leaves kale
- 2 cups of spinach
- 1-2 apples
- 1 cup of grapes
- 1 small piece of ginger

Health Benefit:

Kale is full of powerful antioxidants. It is one of the most nutritious foods out there on the market today. One cup contains about 10% of the RDA of fiber, 9% of calcium and 8% of potassium. Kale has powerful anti-cancer properties as well because it blocks cancer cell growth, and increases DNA repair. It also has anti-inflammatory, cholesterol-lowering, and protective heart and respiratory qualities.

Healing Apple Juice

- 3 medium granny smith apples
- 4 stalks of celery
- 1/2 cup of Kale
- 1 lemon
- 3 cups of spinach

Health Benefit:

Apples are not only delicious and one of my favorite fruits to eat but they are extremely healthy for you. Studies have shown that apples may prevent bone loss; **Alzheimer's, help with asthma, lower cholesterol and may even prevent lung cancer.**

Protein Pack

- 3 cups of spinach
- 1/2 cup of strawberries
- 2 Tbsp. Peanut Butter
- A small piece of ginger
- 1/2 cup of blueberries
- 1 cucumber

Health Benefits:

One cup of spinach has almost 20% of the RDA of dietary fiber, which helps in digestion, prevents constipation, maintains low blood sugar, and curbs overeating. Studies have also shown that the consumption of spinach may also reduce the risk of prostate cancer. I try to put spinach in all my juices because it has so many great health benefits.

Beet Explosion

- 1 large beet
- 1 red apple
- ¼ cup of kale
- 2 cups fresh baby spinach
- 1/2 cup of strawberries
- Spoon full of peanut butter

Health Benefit:

This sweet treat is one of my all-time favorite not only because it's so delicious but because it's so great for my body. Beets are an awesome source of many vitamins and minerals but they also act as nature's Viagra. Yep, you heard it right! The ancient Romans used them medicinally as an aphrodisiac. Who said we need doctors prescribing us with all kinds of pills when nature can provide us with all the healing and medicines we need.

20/20 Vision

- 3 carrots
- 2-3 stalks of celery
- 1/2 cucumber
- 1 green apple
- 1/2 cup of strawberries
- Small piece of ginger

Health Benefit:

Carrots are a crunchy superfood that have many health benefits which include being good for your eyes, helps prevent cancer and promotes healthy skin. Carrots are rich in beta-carotene, the high level of beta-carotene acts as a barrier to cell damage done to the body. It also helps slows down the aging of cells.

Fat Melt

- 1 ½ to 2 cups of baby spinach
- 1 cup of Arugula
- 2 medium Roma tomatoes
- 1 lemon
- 1 small chunk of ginger
- 1 handful of basil
- 1-2 cloves garlic

Health Benefit:

Arugula provides a great source of folate, vitamins A and C, and more than 100 percent of your daily vitamin K needs. Not only is it a great weight-loss food, arugula can also help reduce your risk of bone fracture.

Juice Cleanse

- 1/2 avocado
- 1 green apple
- 1 cup spinach
- 1 handful parsley
- 1/2 cup of kale
- 1/2 cup blue berries

Health Benefit:

Studies have shown that consuming blueberries helps individuals maintain optimal health because they contain vital nutrients the body desperately needs especially since the diets of most Americans today consist of mostly processed foods. Blue berries help improve memory, boost the immune system, improve eye sight and **neutralize free radicals.** These tasty little treats are packed with *Anthocyanin* which is found in the dark blue color of the blueberries. This powerful antioxidant helps neutralize free radicals that can lead to cancer and other diseases.

Grapefruit, Spinach and Strawberry Infusion

- 1 grapefruit
- 2 cups spinach
- 1 handful parsley
- 1/2 cup of strawberries
- 1 green apple
- 1/2 banana

Health Benefit:

There is nothing like a tall glass of cool refreshing grapefruit freshly made from the Ninja blender. This amazing fruit has excellent health benefits because it's rich in vitamin c, it helps lower cholesterol and as a powerful antioxidant, vitamin C protects our bodies against oxidative stress caused by free radical damage and the inflammation associated with asthma and arthritis. Grapefruit is fat free and also contains a high number of fat-burning enzymes. Studies have shown them to also alter insulin levels.

Cholesterol Be Gone

- 1 cup almond milk
- 1/2 cup of oats
- 1 Green apple
- Pinch of cinnamon
- 1/2 cup Blueberries

Health Benefit:

Studies have shown that as little as ½ teaspoon of cinnamon a day can lower your bad cholesterol (LDL). Cinnamon may help treat Type 2 Diabetes by lowering blood sugar levels and increasing the amount of insulin production in the body. Just the scent of cinnamon boosts cognitive function and memory. Cinnamon creates a chemical reaction that when consumed; the body actually reacts chemically to digest the cinnamon. This reaction speeds up the metabolism in order to offset the extra heat that is occurring as a result of the cinnamon. When the metabolism speeds up, you are burning more calories and you will lose weight more quickly.

Omega-3 Special

- 1 small avocado
- 3 cups spinach
- 10 white grapes
- 1 cup of kale
- 1/4 cup flaxseeds
- 1/2 lime
- 1 small piece of ginger

Health Benefit:

Flaxseeds contain omega-3 fatty acids which is great for lowering bad cholesterol. Flaxseeds are also a great source of fiber and work as a natural laxative. Flaxseeds also contain Lignans which may protect against estrogen-dependent cancers such as breast cancer.

Mint Explosion

- 1 avocado
- 1 handful of mint
- 1 cup spinach
- 1 cup parsley
- 1/2 cup of strawberries

Health Benefit:

Avocados are high in beta-sit sterol, a compound that has been shown to lower cholesterol levels. I love to add avocados to most of my juices because they are a great source of protein which is great for muscle recovery after an intense workout.

Almond Joy

- 1 cup almond milk
- 1 Cup of Romaine Lettuce
- 1/2 cup frozen blueberries
- 1/2 cup frozen strawberries
- Pinch of cinnamon
- A scoop of your own favorite protein powder (chocolate)

Health Benefit:

I absolutely love almond milk because it has less cholesterol then regular milk and fewer calories. One cup of almond milk contains only 60 calories, as opposed to 146 calories in whole milk, 122 calories in 2 percent, 102 calories in 1 percent, and 86 calories in skim. It makes for a sweat treat that will help you lose or maintain your current weight.

Lycopene Blast

- 1 tomato
- 1 cup of fresh parsley
- 1 Cup of kale
- 1/2 habanero pepper without seeds
- 1 cup of romaine lettuce
- 1 lemon juice squeezed into blender
- Pinch of cayenne pepper
- 1–2 pinches of flax seeds

Health Benefit:

I like to make this juice when I want something a little on the spicy side, like my grandfather use to tell me when he made his spicy tomato sandwiches, "This tastes so good it will make your tongue slap your brains out" and this juice is sure to do the same. Tomatoes contain vitamins A and C, these vitamins act as an anti-oxidant, working to neutralize dangerous free radicals in the blood stream. Tomatoes also contain lycopene which is one of the most powerful ant-oxidants known to man-kind. Tomatoes can also help repair the damage that smoking does to your body. Tomatoes contain chromogenic acid and coumaric acid, which help to fight against some of the carcinogens brought about by cigarette smoke.

Metabolism Igniter

- 4-6 large leaves of kale with stem
- 1 cup of Green Peppers
- 1/2 handful parsley
- 1/2 cup of cantaloupe
- 1/2 cup of blueberries

Health Benefit:

Not only are green peppers delicious but they are low in calories! You only ingest about 45 calories in one cup. The capsaicin in bell peppers has multiple health benefits. Studies show that green peppers reduce 'bad' cholesterol, control diabetes and provide relief from pain and inflammation.

Daily Glow

- 1 apple
- 1 lemon
- 4 celery stalks
- 2 large carrots
- 6-8 stems parsley
- 6-8 stems fresh mint
- 1/2 banana

Health Benefit:

Mint is great for people who have acne and is sometimes used in facial cleansers for its anti-inflammatory properties and cleansing abilities. Using mint leaves for skin controls oiliness as it contains Vitamin A. It rejuvenates and refreshes the skin making it bright and soft! Consuming mint will be your natural way of getting oil-free naturally glowing skin.

Popeye The Sailor Man

- 1 Whole Spinach Bunch (About 4 cups)
- 2 McIntosh apples
- 1/2 avocado
- 2 oranges
- 1/4 cup Brazil nuts

Health Benefit:

Spinach is packed with an abundance of vitamin K that can prevent the break-down of bones as well as provide nutrient rich protein that is essential for maintaining the strength and density of our bones.

The large quantity of vitamin K in spinach contributes greatly to a healthy nervous system and brain function by providing essential nutrients that keep nerves in the brain healthy and functioning properly.

Fat Eliminator

- 4-6 cups of baby spinach
- 1 lemon, unpeeled
- 2 apples
- 1/2cucumber
- 6 leaves of Romaine
- 1/2 Cup of chia seeds
- Optional: 2-3 garlic cloves

Health Benefit:

There are many health benefits in this juice to mention but probably the most surprising to me where the health benefits of romaine lettuce. I used to think that lettuce had no nutrients in it because I always heard about it being comprised of mostly water but after doing some research I found that nothing could be farther from the truth.

Romaine lettuce is the perfect weight loss food because it is comprised of almost 20 percent protein and it contains large quantities of cellulose and fiber which help fill you up without consuming a lot of calories. Because romaine lettuce has these things it is absolutely awesome when it comes to helping your digestion system. A healthy digestion system is extremely important in helping you maintain weight and remain or get to optimal health since experts suggest that the majority of diseases come from a poor digestion poor digestion system. Rule of thumb, anything vegetable that is green is most likely good for you since these things contain massive amounts of nutrients and healing benefits.

40 Delicious Nutribullet & Ninja Recipes !!!NEW!!

I just bought the Nutribullet a few months back because I wanted to see how it worked compared to the Ninja and I must say I like it indeed. Even though I am a big fan of the Ninja I tend to lean more towards the Nutribullet for the single serving juices and smoothies versus the Ninja. I like to use the Ninja for the big juicing's for several guests, but they both have awesome blending capabilities and are very easy to clean.

Kale & Berry Smoothie Blast

Ingredients

- ½ bananas
- 4 whole strawberries
- 1 handful of kale
- 1 TB honey
- 3 ice cubes
- Sweetened almond milk to the fill line

Health Benefits

The antioxidants and anti-inflammatory properties of kale have made health nuts go crazy over this fantastic leafy superfood; however, kale can be quite bitter and "grassy" in taste. This sweet creamy treat will help you easily consume kale without the bitter taste and it's great for selling your kids on a sweet and tasty treat while at the same time giving those many of their daily needed nutrients.

Green Spinach and Lettuce Smoothie Delight

Makes 2 glasses

Ingredients

- 4 cups chopped romaine lettuce
- 2 cups chopped spinach leaves (about half of a large bunch)
- ½ cup sliced celery
- ½ cup diced apples
- ¼ cup diced pear
- ½ cup sliced banana
- ½ tablespoon fresh lemon juice
- 1 cup of water

Instructions

Wash all vegetables and fruits thoroughly before handling them.

Put romaine lettuce, spinach and water together in a blender on the low setting.

Speed until mixture becomes smooth.

Add celery, apple and pear. Blend mixture at high speed.

Add the banana and lemon juice and puree until well blended.

Pour into glasses and serve fresh.

Variation

Add ½ cup each of parsley and cilantro for an even greener smoothie. Using the stems is okay; chop them so they do not ruin your blender or smoothie maker.

Add an inch of ginger to recipe for an extra sing.

Smoothie info:

This smoothie is designed to help you ingest more greens there for it will assist your body in absorbing more vitamins and minerals plus with all the added fiber it will help keep you full longer.

Green Energizer

Makes 1 glass

Ingredients

- 1 cup fresh spinach
- 1 cup fresh collard greens
- 3 medium sized oranges 3 cups pineapple chunks

Instructions

Squeeze out the juice from the oranges.

Use this fresh juice as liquid base for blending the spinach and collard greens together. Blend at slow speed until smooth.

Add the pineapples to the orange and greens mixture and blend at high speed until well mixed.

Pour and serve

Variation

You can add 6 ice cubes into the mix and blend until smooth.

Smoothie Info

This smoothie is packed with essential vitamins, minerals and proteins that is sure to give you an energy boost. Your body will thank you every time you consume this drink and each time you do you get closer to optimal health.

Papaya Oh My!

Makes 1 glass

- 3 cups spinach leaves
- 2 cups cubed ripe papaya
- 1 cup cubed pear
- 2 tablespoons blue berries
- 8 fresh leaves of mint
- 1 cup of filtered water

Instructions

Pour water into blender. Add papaya first, followed by the pear, berries and mint leaves. Add the spinach last.

Blend on high speed for about 30 seconds or until the smoothie turns into an even and creamy consistency.

Serve Fresh

Variation

You can replace the papaya with a whole banana which makes for a delicious sweet and creamy smoothie.

Smoothie Info

This smoothie recipe has plenty of protein, folate, magnesium and potassium. It's also high in vitamins A, B1, B6, C and K which is excellent for the skin and eyes.

Pina Colada Smoothie Delight

Ingredients

- 1 cup chopped spinach
- 4 cups fresh ripe pineapple chunks
- ½ cup shredded coconut meat
- 4 tablespoons dried pitted dates
- 2 cups unsweetened coconut water
- 2 cups unsweetened coconut water
- 2 cups ice cubes

Instructions

Put all ingredients in a blender. Remember to put the liquid first and the greens last. Add ingredients in between.

Blend on high speed until a creamy and smooth puree is achieved.

Pour into glasses and serve.

Variation

For a creamier taste you can even add 3 tablespoons of raw cashew nuts to this recipe.

Smoothie Info

Spinach is said to be one of the most powerful antioxidants known to humans. This wonderful green is packed with nutrients that prevent horrible diseases like dementia because it has folate, vitamin E, and vitamin K.

Kiwi Health Blast

Makes 1 glass

Ingredients

- 1 cup chopped spinach leaves
- 1 cup chopped kale leaves
- 1 cup chopped Swiss chard leaves
- ½ cup sliced ripe bananas
- ½ kiwi fruit
- Juice of ½ lemons
- 1 cup distilled water
- 1 teaspoon bee pollen
- ½ teaspoon maca powder

Instructions

Wash all ingredients thoroughly.

Prepare as directed in the recipe.

Put all ingredients in a blender. Blend at high speed until smooth.

Pour into a glass and serve immediately

Replace water with same amount of unsweetened coconut water for extra alkaline in your green smoothie.

If kiwis aren't in season, substitute it with mango or papaya.

Minty Smoothie Blast

Makes 2 glasses

Ingredients

- 1 cup chopped kale leaves
- 10 pieces mint leaves
- 2 whole pitted dates
- 2 tablespoons raw cashew butter
- 1 ½ cups distilled water

Instructions

Put all ingredients in a blender. Blend on high speed until smooth.

Pour into glasses and serve immediately

Variation

Substitute pitted dates with 1 tablespoon of raw coconut nectar or raw agave nectar.

Smoothie Fact

Mint is not only good for freshening your breath but it also aids in digestion and helps to sooth nausea and headaches.

Avocado Lime Weight Loss Extravaganza

Ingredients

- 1 cup young spinach leaves
- ½ cup sliced cucumber
- ½ avocado fruit
- 2 whole limes
- Sweetener (honey, agave or stevia) to taste
- 6 pieces ice cubes

Instructions

Wash vegetables and fruits thoroughly.

Take out the leaves of the spinach and discard stems.

Without peeling, cut cucumber into half-inch slices.

Remove see of avocado. Using a spoon, scoop out flesh from the peeling.

Peel and quarter limes

In a blender, place cucumber, avocado, spinach and lime. Add ice cubes and desired amount of sweetener.

Blend all ingredients until smooth.

Pour into a glass and drink fresh.

Variation

Add ½ teaspoon cinnamon powder to add some kick to your smoothie.

If you find your smoothie too thick, add ½ cup of cold distilled water and blend again before serving.

Smoothie Info

Limes are especially good for women's health. The citrus gems contain calcium and folate, two nutrients that are vital for post-menopausal women and women of child bearing age. Limes are also anti-carcinogenic and can help prevent the formation of kidney stones. Limes may even lower cholesterol.

Kale Health Optimizer

Makes 1 glass

Ingredients

- 1 cup kale leaves
- 1 medium sized Granny Smith apple
- 1 medium sized avocado
- ¼ lemon fruit
- 1 tablespoon sliced ginger
- A pinch of salt
- ½ cup distilled water

Instructions

Rinse kale in running water. Tear leaves apart.

Without peeling, core and separate apples.

Cut avocado into halves, remove seed and scoop out flesh using a tablespoon.

Peel lemon and remove seeds.

Peel ginger and cut into thin slices.

Put all ingredients in a blender.

Blend on high speed until well mixed and smooth Pour into a small glass and enjoy

Variation

Use limes instead of lemon for a slightly different taste.

Instead of adding sweetener like honey agave nectar, you can make this smoothie taste sweeter by adding more apples.

Instead of avocado, you can also use equal part banana in this recipe.

Smoothie info

Kale is another great superfood that is sure to help change your life by changing your health. Kale is full of chlorophyll which helps purify the blood. It also helps boost your immune system and clear lung and intestinal congestion.

Watermelon Smoothie Delight

Ingredients

- 8 leaves of mint
- 8 leaves of sweet basil
- 8 leaves of coriander
- 2 cups watermelon chunks
- ½ small avocado fruit
- ½ cup cucumber slices
- Juice of ½ lime fruit
- ½ cup distilled water

Instructions

Remove seeds from watermelon before cutting into chunks. Scoop out flesh from the avocado fruit. Slice cucumbers into half-inch thickness.

Put all ingredients in a blender in this order: mint, basil, coriander, water, watermelon, avocado, cucumber, lime juice. Blend on high speed until smooth.

Pour into a tall glass and serve.

Variation

Add ½ teaspoon of fennel seeds and ½ cup oats for a more filling version of this smoothie.

Put smoothie inside the freezer to cool it down for a few minutes before serving.

Smoothie Info

The health benefits of cucumber and watermelon are plentiful. Watermelons are mostly water, about 90 percent but this amazing fruit is filled with nutrients such as b6 and c, lots of lycopene, antioxidants and amino acids. There is even a small amount of potassium.

The health benefits of cucumber includes antioxidants, helps skin with its plethora of vitamins and minerals such as magnesium, potassium and silicon. Cucumber also aids in weight loss and cuts down your chances of getting certain cancers.

Apple Detox Smoothie

Makes 2 Glasses

Ingredients

- 1 cup shredded romaine lettuce
- ½ cup broccoli heads
- 1 medium sized apple
- ½ orange
- ½ cup distilled water
- 1 cup ice cubes

Instructions

Rinse greens under running water.

Peel and core apple. Cut into 1 inch cubes.

Peel orange. Remove seeds and separate into segments

Put all ingredients in a blender. Blend on high speed until thoroughly combined.

Pour into a glass and serve.

Variation

Add 1 tablespoon of chopped parsley into the mix for added kick.

Smoothie Fact

You have made and excellent health choice not only by purchasing this eBook which is full of recipes that will surely assist you in getting to optimal health but this particular smoothie is full of fiber, minerals, vitamins and phytochemicals that will assist in getting rid of toxins in the body.

Fig and Ginger Twist Smoothie

Makes 1 glass

Ingredients

- 1 cup spinach
- 1 cup figs (about 4 medium sized fruits)
- ½ tablespoon chopped ginger
- 2 whole pitted dates (pre-soaked)
- ½ cup distilled water
- 1 cup ice cubes

Instructions

In a blender, add spinach and water. Blend until smooth.

Add all remaining ingredients and process until blended smooth.

Pour into a glass and enjoy.

Variation

Add a tablespoon of flaxseeds for adding some kick.

Smoothie Info

Figs are a good source of potassium and minerals that helps control blood pressure. Fig is also a sweet way to lose weight being that they are a good source of dietary fiber. Studies have shown that postmenopausal women have had a reduction in breast cancer risk for those consuming the most fruit fiber compared to those eating less fiber and the Fig is a great fruit filled with the fiber one needs throughout the day.

Banana Smoothie Delight

Makes 1 glass

Ingredients

- 1 cup chopped kale leaves
- 2 cups diced ripe bananas
- ½ cup distilled water
- ½ cup ice cubes

Instructions

Rinse kale in running water and clean thoroughly.

Peel bananas and cut into 1-inch slices

Put all ingredients in a blender and blend until smooth.

Pour into a glass and enjoy.

Variation

For a sweeter taste, add 1 piece of apple (cored and cut into wedges) into the recipe. This will infuse your smoothie with the toxin removal properties of apples.

Smoothie Info

Bananas are Americas' favorite fresh fruit. This wonderful food is high in potassium and pectin; they can also be a great way to get magnesium and vitamins C and B6. Bananas are high in antioxidants, which can provide protection from free radicals.

Mean Green Machine Smoothie

1 Glass

Ingredients

- 2 pieces apples
- ½ a banana
- ½ piece cucumber
- 1 cup water

Instructions

Peel, core and cut apples into 1-inch cubes.

Peel banana and cut into 1 inch slices.

Without peeling, cut cucumbers into 1-inch cubes.

Place all ingredients in a blender and blend until smooth.

Pour into a glass and serve right away!

Variation

To make a cold smoothie, use only ½ cup of water and add ½ cup of ice cubes. Blend well.

Smoothie Info

A study shows that drinking apple juice could keep Alzheimer's away and fight the effects of aging on the brain, people who eat fruits and other high-fiber foods also gain some amount of protection against Parkinson's. Apples could also reduce your risk of developing pancreatic cancer and other cancers. Keep eating those apples!

Chocolate Green Machine Smoothie

Makes 1 glass

Ingredients

- ½ cup chopped kale leaves
- 1 cup chopped romaine lettuce leaves
- ½ cup Swiss chard
- 1 cup sliced ripe bananas
- 1 teaspoon unsweetened cacao powder
- 1 tablespoon natural honey
- 1 cup unsweetened coconut water

Instructions

Rinse and prepare greens and fruits.

Peel bananas and cut into 1 inch slices.

Put all ingredients in a blender and process until smooth.

Pour into a glass and serve immediately.

Variation

Add juice of ½ lemons for extra zest.

Smoothie Info

Cacao beans are seeds of the Theobromine cacao tree. They have chemicals called flavonoids, a type of antioxidant compound that promotes general health and might even lower risk for several diseases.

Green Giant Smoothie

Makes 1 glass

Ingredients

- 1 cup chopped kale leaves
- ½ cup Brussels sprouts
- ½ cup spinach leaves
- ½ avocado
- 1 medium sized green apple
- ½ cup filtered water
- ½ cup ice cubes

Instructions

Wash and prepare the greens

Scoop out the avocado flesh. Discard the seed.

Without peeling, core the apple and cut into 1-inch cubes.

In a blender, mix kale, Brussels sprouts, spinach and filtered water until smooth.

Add avocado, apple and ice cubes. Blend until smooth.

Variation

Add 1 teaspoon chia seeds for an added crunch

Add ½ cup broccoli or clover sprouts for extra greens

Smoothie Info

Brussels sprouts are rich in many nutrients. They have a great source of vitamin C and vitamin K. They also have an excellent source of other nutrients including folate, manganese, vitamin B6 dietary fiber, choline, copper, vitamin B1 and many other health benefits.

Pineapple Twist

Makes 1 glass

Ingredients

- ½ cup of fresh pineapple chunks
- 2 tbsps. granulated sugar
- ¼ teaspoon iodized salt
- 1 cup filtered water

Instructions

Mix sugar and salt in a cup of water, stir until melted.

Put pineapple chunks in sugar and salt water and soak for 8 minutes

Pour pineapple and water in a juicer and run juicer on high speed for 30 seconds.

Pour juice into a glass and drink fresh.

Variation

For a thicker and cooler alternative, add ½ cup crushed ice to pineapple and water mixture before running the juicer.

Add 2-3 mint leaves to the recipe for extra flavor.

Health Benefit

This delicious juice is an awesome fat eliminator because pineapples aid in digestion and help get rid of inflammation in the body by ridding the stomach and intestines of fat. Pineapples are also an awesome source of vitamin C, which gives protection from the flu.

Sweet Guava

Makes 1 glass

Ingredients

- 1 whole medium ripe guava
- ½ cup cold distilled water
- 2 tablespoons honey

Instructions

Wash guava and cut into halves.

Remove seed core and cut into 2-inch pieces.

Process guava and cold water in a juicer.

Mix honey in guava juice. Drink immediately.

Instructions

Use natural, unprocessed honey for better health benefits. Add honey to taste.

Health Benefit

Guava is great for weight loss because it has very little calories and it's delicious and packed full of fiber.

Banana Health Blast

Makes 1 glass

Ingredients

- 8 whole strawberries
- 2 medium sized ripe bananas

Instructions

Take off leaves and stems from the strawberries

Peel bananas and cut into 2-inch slices.

Put everything into the juicer and enjoy!

Variation

Add crushed ice before running in the juicer, this will make for a deliciously cold treat.

Add 10 pieces of pitted dates into the recipe for extra punch in taste.

For a sweeter taste, add 1 piece apple (cored and cut into wedges) into the

Recipe. This will also infuse your juice with the toxin removal properties of apples.

Health Benefit

Strawberries are high in antioxidants, which slows the aging process by blocking free radicals from the body's system.

Bananas are high in resistant starch, a type of fiber found in carbohydrate-rich foods that enhances fat burning.

Pomegranate explosion

Makes 1 glass

Ingredients

- 1 cup lychee
- ½ whole pomegranates
- 1 teaspoon food-grade vanilla essence

Instructions

Remove skin and seeds from lychees.

Peel Pomegranate and slice into 1-inch cubes.

Process lychees pomegranate and vanilla essence in a blender until mixed well.

Pour into a glass and drink fresh.

Variation

Throw in some crushed ice before blending ingredients together to make a refreshing smoothie.

Health Benefits

Lychees are low in cholesterol, saturated fats and sodium but they are high in copper, potassium, Vitamin C and dietary fiber.

Pomegranate is considered by health experts as a super fruit when it comes to weight loss. It contains massive amounts of vitamins and minerals that help detoxify the entire body, making you more vibrant and energetic. This amazing fruit also helps cut down on heart disease by preventing the harmful cholesterol buildup in ones arteries. You will also attain healthier more glowing skin complexion that is sure to make the prettiest person you know jealous.

Mango Paradise

Makes 2 glasses

Ingredients

- ½ small watermelons
- 1 whole ripe mango
- 1 ½ cup fresh pineapple chunks

Instructions

Remove the green outer rind from the watermelon. Slice the watermelon into 2-inch chunks.

Peel the mango and cut away the inner seed from the flesh. Cut flesh into 2-inch slices.

Process mango, watermelon and pineapple together in a juicer.

Chill juice for half an hour, then serve over ice.

Variation

Add one cup of cold filtered water to the juice to thin its consistency. Adding water will yield to three glasses of juice.

Health benefits

Watermelon is cholesterol-free, high in water content, low in sodium and extremely rich in ant-cancer phytochemical lycopene. Watermelon's high water content will help muscles become hydrated which will intern help reduce muscle fatigue.

Muskmelon Heaven

Makes 1 glass

Ingredients

- 10 whole loquats
- 1 small wedge of muskmelon
- 2/3 cups fresh pineapple chunks
- 2 tablespoons honey
- ½ cup cold distilled water

Instructions

Wash loquat and remove skin. Cut into 1-inch pieces.

Remove outer rind and seeds from muskmelon. Cut into 2-inch slices.

Process loquat, muskmelon, pineapple and water in a juicer for 15 seconds.

Pour into a glass.

Add honey and stir until fully dissolved into the juice. Drink fresh.

Variation

Serve chilled or over crushed ice for a refreshing drink during those hot spring and summer days and nights!

Substitute pineapple and honey with one whole red apple and one whole lemon for a citrusy, less sweet taste.

Health Benefit

The combined superfoods of the fruits loquat and muskmelon makes this juice a potent mix for removing fat around the mid-section and reducing cellulite around your hip thighs and buttocks.

Muskmelon has a plethora of beta-carotene, sodium, magnesium, potassium and vitamins A, B and C. It has large sums of dietary fiber and has zero cholesterol. Muskmelon also has a sweet taste, which can make any boring diet more bearable.

Papaya Passion

Makes 1 glass

Ingredients

- 1 small papaya
- 1 whole red apple
- 5 whole pitted dates

Instructions

Wash skin and remove the seeds of the papaya. Cut into 2-inch slices.

Wash and core pineapples. Slice into wedges.

Put all ingredients in a juicer or blender until a smooth juice is made.

Drink chilled or over ice cubes.

Variation

Add a teaspoon of finely chopped mint leaves to juice before drinking to add a burst of color in your juice and to make it more refreshing.

Dilute the juice with ¼ cup lime juice instead of water to further enhance the taste of papaya.

Health Benefit

Papaya is packed full of vitamins A and C, calcium, iron, niacin, potassium, riboflavin and thiamin, it's also low in calories and full of energy sustaining compounds.

Muskmelon and Apple Delight

Makes 1 glass

Ingredients

- 1 small wedge muskmelon
- 1 whole red apple
- 1 whole lemon
- ½ cup ice cubes

Instructions

Skin muskmelon and remove the seeds. Cut into 2-inch slices.

Wash, peel and core apples. Cut into 1-inch slices.

Peel lemon and remove seeds. Cut into half-inch slices.

Process muskmelon, apple, lemon and ice cubes in a juicer until a smooth juice is made.

Serve and drink right away.

Variation

Add a dash of cinnamon or cayenne pepper to help give your metabolism a boost.

Health Benefit

The presence of muskmelon and lemon helps ease symptoms of high blood pressure and regulates sugar absorption.

Sione Michelson

Fruit-topic

Makes 1 glass

Ingredients

- 2 medium red apples
- 4 whole kiwis
- 2 medium oranges
- 1 medium pineapple

Instructions

Core apples and slice into wedges.

Peel the kiwis. Cut into one-inch thick slices

Remove the outer rind of the oranges but try to leave all the white skin since it has lots of nutrients.

Be sure to removes seeds since this has a potential for making you sick.

Peel core and cut pineapple into spears.

Remove the outer rind of the lemons and lime quarters.

Run all ingredients into juicer. Stir and shake before serving.

Variation

Add ¼ lemons fruit and another ¼ lime into the recipe to make your juice more tangy and citrusy. Remember that adding fresh lemons to your juice will help increase your chances for weight loss because of the citric acid in the lemons helps kick the body's metabolism into high gear.

Health Benefits

Apples are an excellent source of pectin which is an enzyme that removes toxins from the intestines.

Oranges are filled with Vitamin C which helps reduce your chances of catching a cold. Oranges also help relieve constipation and inhibits kidney ailments.

Kiwis are rich in antioxidants and strengthen the immune system. Kiwis contain more Vitamin C than oranges, as much potassium as bananas and high levels of appetite-suppressing fibers.

Grape & Cactus Delight

Makes 1 glass

Ingredients

- 1 cup seedless grapes
- ¼ cup cactus pear fruit juice
- 2 small wedges of muskmelon
- 2 whole medium ripe mangoes
- ½ cup ice cubes

Instructions

Wash grapes thoroughly.

Skin muskmelon and remove all the seeds. Cut into 2-inch slices

Peel mango and cut away the seed from the flesh. Cut flesh into 2 inch slices.

Put all ingredients, including cactus juice and ice cubes, in a juicer. Enjoy.

Variation

If you cannot find seedless grapes, don't worry. You can juice whole grapes with seeds intact for additional antioxidant properties derived from grape seeds.

Use 2 whole, skinned fresh cactus pear fruit in place of fruit juice indicated in this recipe to get more raw fiber from the fruit.

Health Benefits

Grapes have a plethora of health benefits aside from losing weight. They are also packed with Vitamin C, boost energy, improve vision and inhibit the growth of cancer cells.

Cactus pear fruit (also called prickly pear) is an excellent appetite suppressant because it is rich in dietary fiber that will make you feel full. The fruit also lowers blood pressure and improves the health of the vascular system.

Beet & Celery Delight

Makes 1 glass

Ingredients

- ½ cup of cubed beets or 1 small whole beet.
- 1 cup celery stalks (about 5 stalks), chopped.
- 1 cup of spinach leaves chopped.
- ¼ cup of coriander leaves (about 2 sprigs), chopped
- 1 teaspoon salt

Instructions

Rinse celery, spinach and coriander in running water. Chop

Wash beets and cut into wedges.

Process all ingredients in a juicer. Pour in a glass and drink fresh.

Variation

Add a squeeze of lemon in your juice for a tangy experience.

Health Benefit

Beets are an excellent source of nutrients and are powerful detoxifier of the bladder, kidney and liver.

Celery is high in fiber, low in cholesterol and low in protein- an excellent weight loss veggie!

Cucumber & Kale Explosion

Makes 1 glass

Ingredients

- 2 whole small cucumbers
- ½ cup kale
- ¼ cup spinach
- ¼ cup parsley
- ¼ cup Swiss chard
- ½ slice lemon

Instructions

Rinse Kale, spinach, parsley and Swiss chard under cold running water. Without removing small stems, chop each vegetable separately.

Wash cucumbers and slice into 1 inch chunks.

Remove rind and seeds from lemon. Slice thinly.

Run all ingredients through a juicer. Pour into a glass and serve fresh.

Variation

Add a natural sweetener like stevia if you want to improve the taste of this mean green health juice.

It is best to drink vegetable juices at room temperature to preserve nutrients that may dissolve at colder temperature. If you should want to have this juice cold, pour juice over ice cubes just before drinking. Do not chill.

Health Benefit

Kale contains more calcium than milk, more iron than beef and ten times more Vitamin C than spinach.

Sione Michelson

All green vegetables effectively clean the digestive tract and the blood. Green juices are especially effective at giving people more energy as it also cleanses your body.

Asparagus Delight

Makes 1 glass

Ingredients

- 1/3 cup asparagus in cold running water. Cut into 1-inch cubes.

Boil 2 cups water and add asparagus. Cook until it becomes tender. Do not cook until it's mushy or olive green in color. Remove asparagus from water and dry. Set aside.

Rinse coriander in cold running water. Chop coriander leaves

Wash onions. Chop into 1- inch cubes.

Put asparagus, coriander and onion in a juicer. Add 1 ½ cup distilled water and sugar. Process until a smooth juice is produced.

Pour into a glass and drink fresh.

Variation

Squeeze a few drops of lemon to counter the strong taste of coriander.

For an added kick, add 4 thin slices of ginger before juicing.

Health Benefit

Asparagus is an alkaline based vegetable which makes it ideal for burning fat. It is low in calories but high in protein, folic acid, beta-carotene and Vitamin C.

Coriander leaves contain a host of nutrients, fiber, carbohydrates, vitamin C and minerals such as calcium, iron, niacin, potassium, phosphorous, riboflavin, thiamin and oxalic acid. Coriander promotes digestion and cleanses and strengthens the stomach. It is also a good diuretic (promotes the production of urine), which helps rid the body of toxins.

Splendid Carrot Juice

Makes 1 glass

Ingredients

- 2 medium carrots
- 1 cup watercress (about 15 sprigs)
- ½ cup spinach leaves
- ¼ cup coriander leaves (about 3 sprigs)
- 2 whole tomatoes

Instructions

Add 1 teaspoon of ground black pepper and 1 teaspoon of rock salt before juicing for an added kick.

Health Benefit

Carrots are high in polyunsaturated fats or good cholesterol. Carrots are also rich in fiber, which helps speed up the body's metabolism and prevents it from storing energy as fat.

Watercress is great source potassium, which serves as a diuretic to draw excess fluid from the body. Because watercress has more Sulphur than almost any other vegetable, it is excellent in the blood purification, protein absorption, cell building and promoting healthy skin and hair.

When consumed raw, spinach is an excellent source of foliate, manganese and vitamins A and K. Spinach is high in fiber and low in fat, sodium cholesterol and protein.

Broccoli Special

Makes 1 glass

Ingredients

- 3 cups broccoli (about 2 stalks)
- ½ cup chopped green bell pepper (about ½ medium whole)
- 2 cups carrots (about 4 medium whole)

Instructions

Rinse broccoli in cold running water. Cut into 2-inch pieces.

Wash bell peppers, remove seeds and chop.

Wash carrots, remove tops and cut into 2-inch slices.

Juice the broccoli, bell pepper and carrots together. Serve right away.

Variation:

Carrots are the most versatile vegetable that can be used in making healthy Juices. You can combine them with almost any vegetable or fruit and it will still taste good. Try adding a small apple into this recipe to make a sweet concoction.

Health Benefits

Rich in folate, manganese and vitamins A and K, broccoli is an excellent vegetable for losing weight because it is high in fiber and very low in cholesterol. You can help yourself with almost an unlimited serving of raw broccoli and you will feel satisfied without having to gain hard-to-burn calories!

Unknown too many, bell peppers are actually a good source of lycopene, beta carotene, potassium and fiber. Bell pepper increases your metabolism, controls your appetite and suppresses your craving for sweets.

Carrots are an excellent source of beta carotene, calcium, iron, magnesium, potassium, riboflavin and vitamins A and C.

Cabbage and Beet Delight

Makes 1 glass

Ingredients

- 2 large leaves of cabbage
- 1 small beet
- ½ medium cucumbers
- 4 medium carrots

Instructions

Wash all ingredients thoroughly

Roll cabbage leaves tightly into balls

Peel beet and cut into cubes

Cut cucumber into cubes

Peel carrots and slice into chunks.

Process all ingredients in a juicer. Drink Fresh!

Variation

Use more cucumber if you want to increase the quantity of your juice. Adding water will do the same trick, but using water-rich cucumber instead will add in more nutrients than water.

Juicing Tip:

When using cabbages in a recipe, you will extract more juice from the cabbage if you run it with hard produce like beets.

Health Benefits

Cabbages are extremely high in Vitamin K manganese. Those on high-fiber, low-fat, and low-sodium and low protein weight loss program will benefit most from incorporating cabbages into their diet.

Fruit and Veggie Extravaganza

Makes 1 glass

Ingredients

- 5 whole oranges
- ½ cup parsley

Instructions

Peel oranges and remove the seeds

Rinse parsley in running water, Leave for a few minutes to dry before chopping.

Put oranges and parsley through a juicer. Pour into a chilled glass and drink immediately.

Variation

For a fancy presentation, form two layers when pouring this juice into a glass by juicing the oranges and the parsley separately. Pour the orange juice first and then slowly pour parsley juice over it. The parsley juice will not mix with the orange juice and keep its place above it in your glass. You can just stir the juice before drinking if you do not enjoy the taste of pure parsley.

Juicing Tip

When Juicing oranges, remember to remove the outer rind but leave as much white skin intact as these are rich in nutrients.

Health Benefits

Herbs such as parsley figure well in a weight loss program because they aid in digesting and absorbing foo while providing a low-calorie diet.

Apple & Carrot Delight

Makes 1 glass

Ingredients

- 2 medium apples
- 3 medium carrots
- 4 Large stalks of celery

Instructions

Wash all Ingredients thoroughly

Core the apples but do not peel. Cut into segments.

Remove greens from the carrots. Slice into 1-inch cubes.

Cut celery into 2-inch sticks

Run all ingredients through a juicer. Pour into a glass and drink.

Variation

Add a dash of cinnamon to the juice and stir before serving for an added kick.

For added natural sweetness, put in one or more apple to your juice.

Health Benefits

This recipe is good for those who are still easing themselves into juicing and are not quite prepared for dark colored juices- you get all the benefits from the fresh and healthy ingredients without feeling "hardcore" about it.

Pear & Celery Delight

Makes 1 glass

Ingredients

- ½ cube pear slices (or 1 medium fruit)
- ½ cup diced celery (or 1 large stalk)
- 1-inch cube of ginger root

Instructions

Make sure all ingredients are thoroughly washed before preparing according to measurement indicated.

Run all ingredients through a blender. Pour over ice cubes in a glass and serve immediately.

Variation

For a creamier texture to this juice, process juice and ice cubes (about 5 pieces) in a blender.

Health Benefits

Pears act as a mild laxative while celery is a good natural diuretic. On top of this, ginger aids in proper digestion.

Banana & Apple Delight

Makes 1 glass

Ingredients

- 2/3 cup sliced bananas
- 2/3 cup sliced raw bitter melon
- 2/3 cup diced apples
- ½ cup distilled water

Instructions

Wash and then prepare or cut bananas, apples and bitter melon according to recipe specification.

Process all ingredients in the juicer. Pour into a glass and serve immediately.

Variation

Try adding a teaspoon of vinegar to the recipe to prevent color darkening of banana and apple due to oxidation.

If you still find the juice to be bitter despite the apple in the recipe, add a tablespoon or two of the natural honey to sweeten it more.

Health Benefits

Bitter melon aids in digestion and detoxification. It also helps regulate energy and fat storage.

Mango & Peach Surprise

Makes 1 glass

Ingredients

- ¼ cup mangoes
- 1 medium ripe banana
- ¼ cup peaches
- ¼ cup spinach
- ¼ cup distilled water

Instructions

Peel mangoes and separate the flesh from the seed. Cut flesh into 2-inch cubes

Peel bananas. Cut into 2-inch slices.

Cut peaches in half. Scoop out the flesh.

Rinse spinach in cold running water. Chop

Process all ingredients, including the water, in a juicer or a blender.

Pour juice over crushed ice in a glass. Drink immediately.

Variation

Chop 3 fresh mint leaves and add in the juice for a more refreshing treat.

Juicing Tip

The base ingredient in this juice is banana. Try it with any fruit and vegetable combination-like strawberries, pineapples, kale, Swiss chard or lettuce.

If you want a creamier juice, try adding avocados or coconut.

Sione Michelson

This juice is best taken as your breakfast, so if you are constantly in a rush in the morning, you can prepare this juice in the evening and just put it in the refrigerator. Juices and smoothies will usually remain fresh for 24 hours.

Health Benefits

Aside from potassium, bananas are also rich in fiber, amino acids, manganese and Vitamin B6. It is an excellent fat burning food due to its high content of resistant starch, which helps rid the body of excess fats.

Orange & Beet Treat

Makes 1 glass

Ingredients

- 2 oranges
- 1 medium sized red beet
- 4 medium sized carrots
- 8 pieces mint leaves

Instructions

Wash all ingredients thoroughly, especially the beets.

Peel oranges and remove seeds, but leave as much white pith as possible to retain fiber.

Remove greens from the beets. You may or may not peel the beets before cutting into 1-inch cubes.

Process all ingredients in a juicer. Pour into a glass and serve.

Variation

Add 2 medium stalks of celery to the recipe to further enhance the taste of the beets.

Juicing Tip

When a recipe calls for juicing vegetables and fruits with their peel or skin intact (such as beets and carrots), it is best to use organic produce since they are grown without the use of chemical fertilizers or pesticides.

Health Benefit

This juice is a powerful antioxidant. Although best to take in moderation, beets are good for weight loss because they are low in fat, fight water retention and help your body flush out toxins.

Pineapple, Carrot, & Lime Delight

Makes 1 glass

Ingredients

- 1 cup pineapple chunks
- 1 cup chopped carrots
- 1 tablespoon lime juice
- ½ small red or green chili
- 4-5 ice cubes

Instructions

Make sure all produce were washed thoroughly before chopping or juicing.

Prepare pineapples and carrots according to cut and measurement required by the recipe.

Slice the chili in half and remove seeds and stem.

Juice the pineapple and carrot juice, lime juice chili and ice cubes in a blender. Consume immediately.

Variation

For a more pulpy juice, skip juicing the pineapple and carrots separately and process all ingredients at once using a blender.

Health Benefits

This is a Vitamin C packed juice that will help boost your immune system.

Adding chilies to your juice not only gives a surprising kick but also helps in accelerating your metabolism.

Kiwi, Pineapple & Broccoli Delight

Makes 1 glass

Ingredients

- 1 whole kiwi, peeled and sliced
- 2/3 cup pineapple chunks
- 1/3 cup cucumber slices
- 1/3 cup diced broccoli

Instructions

Carefully wash and prepare all ingredients according to the recipe.

Run everything through a juicer. Pour into a glass and serve.

Variation

Add 1/3 cup crushed ice to the juice and stir before serving for an awesomely refreshing drink.

Health Benefits

Pineapples are rich in enzymes that will help detoxify the body by flushing out mucus build-up

Lemon & Apple Delight

Makes 1 glass

Ingredients

- 1 green apple
- ½ lemon fruit
- 5 outer leaves of red leaf lettuce
- 1 cucumber

Instructions

Wash all ingredients thoroughly.

Core apple and slice into wedges.

Peel lemon and remove the seeds.

Shred red leaf lettuce into salad size servings.

Slice cucumber into 2-inch pieces.

Process all ingredients in a juicer or blender. Serve over crushed ice if you prefer your juice cold.

Variation

Add ½ small ginger (peeled and chopped) for an extra zing to this juice.

Juicing tip

Red leaf lettuce will make your juice deep green in color with a smoother taste compared to bitter alternatives such as kale, spinach and parsley.

When incorporating ginger in your juice, expect to feel a slight burn in your body-that's ginger rousing your blood circulation and jumpstarting your body's immune system!

Health Benefit

Red leaf lettuce is rich in calcium, folate, iron and vitamins A and K.

Using ginger in your juice will not only give a spicy and citrusy taste; it will also help boost your immune system by shielding your body from viral infections and inflammatory conditions such as arthritis. Ginger also stimulates sweating which is important in discharging toxins through the skin.

Cucumber & Apple Delight

Makes 1 glass

Ingredients

- 4 red apples
- 1 small cucumber
- 2 large carrots
- 2 celery stalks

Instructions

Wash all ingredients thoroughly. Pay particular attention to the carrots, which tend to bind dirt and soil in their skin.

Core the apples but do not remove the outer skin. Cut into wedges.

Without peeling, cut cucumber, carrots and celery into 3-inch strips.

Process all ingredients in a juicer. Best served over crushed ice.

Variation

Use a medium sized cucumber to increase the yield of this recipe.

Health Benefit

This delicious juice is ideal for flushing out toxins and unwanted fats from the body.

Apple & Kale Special

Makes 1 glass

Ingredients

- 1 medium red apple
- 3 large leaves of kale
- 2 large leaves of lettuce
- 3 stalks of celery
- ½ medium cucumbers

Instructions

Wash all ingredients thoroughly.

Core apple but do not peel.

Cut celery into 2-inch lengths

Roll kale and lettuce leaves into balls and run together with apple or celery through a juicer. Add the cucumber chunks to juice together with the previous four ingredients.

Pour into a glass and enjoy this delicious green juice.

Variation

Add a small piece of peeled ginger for extra zing to your juice.

Health Benefits

The combination of kale, lettuce, celery and apple makes this juice a great cleansing juice that will help rid your body of toxins and unhealthy fats.

Carrot & Apple Health Craze

Makes 1 glass

Ingredients

- 2 cups chopped carrots (about 4 medium wholes)
- 1 cup quartered apple (or 1 small whole)
- 2 cups spinach leaves
- 2 stalks of celery (10 inch long each)
- 4 parsley leaves

Instructions

Rinse all ingredients in running water.

Remove greens and chop the carrots into 1-inch chunks.

Without peeling, core and quarter the apple

Roll spinach leaves into small balls that would fit into the feeding chute of your juicer.

Juice a chunk of carrot with spinach and parsley leaves. This process will help extract more juice from greens.

Juice celery stalks and then the apples.

Pour into a drinking glass and serve.

Add one small cucumber to this recipe to increase the quantity of your juice per serving.

If strawberries are in season, add 5 strawberries to the recipe. Strawberries, which go well with spinach, will help enhance the flavor of this juice. Drinking the juice of carrot and parsley will help you trim your food cravings because these vegetables are appetite suppressants.

Grape, Apple & Red Cabbage Flavorific

Makes 1 glass

Ingredients

- 1 cup seedless grapes
- 1 1/3 cup chopped apples
- ¼ cup coarsely chopped red cabbage
- 3 large stalks of celery
- 1 thumb of ginger
- 1 tablespoon balsamic vinegar

Instruction

Wash all ingredients thoroughly

Core and chop apples into 1 inch cubes. Chop red cabbage. Peel ginger and slice into strips.

Run all fruits and vegetables through a juicer. Pour into a glass.

Add balsamic vinegar and stir before drinking.

Variation

Add the juice of half a lemon fruit to recipe for a sweet citrusy taste to counteract the acidity of the balsamic vinegar.

Health Benefit

Don't let this purple colored juice fool you-it is packed with an excellent amount of vitamins and nutrients that is as healthy green as any power fruit and vegetable juice.

Just like your green cabbage, variety, red cabbage is rich in lactic acid, phytonutrients and vitamins A, C and E- but that's not all. Unlike its green sister, red cabbage derives its color from anthocyanin, an antioxidant that counteracts obesity-causing metabolic syndrome, insulin problems and hypertension. Anthocyanin also helps protect brain cells from Alzheimer's disease.

Sione Michelson

Apple & Beet-Sweet Potato Treat

Makes 1 glass

Ingredients

- 2 medium red apples
- 2 medium beets
- 1 cup sweet potatoes cubes (about one 5 inch long potato)
- 1 medium red bell pepper
- 1 large carrot.

Instructions

Wash all ingredients thoroughly.

Core apple and remove seeds. Cut into 1-inch cubes.

Cut beets into wedges.

Wash bell peppers, remove seeds and cut into half-inch strips lengthwise.

Remove greens and chop the carrot into 1-inch cubes.

Run all ingredients through a juicer. Pour into a glass. Stir before serving.

Variation

Add 1 medium sized orange to the recipe for a citrusy flavor to your juice. Remember to peel the orange and remove its seeds before juicing.

Health Benefits

Sweet potatoes are high in dietary fiber, high in water content, low in calories and low in sugar. It is thus an excellent addition to you weight loss diet.

40 Delicious Smoothie Recipes

SMOOTHIES

Morning Coffee Delight

Ingredients

- One banana peeled
- 1 tablespoon of chia seeds (soak them for at least five minutes)
- ½ teaspoon of Vanilla Extract (vanilla protein powder can be substituted)
- 1 Cup coconut milk (unsweetened)
- 5 Strawberries (Medium to Large)
- ½ teaspoon instant coffee grounds

Instructions

Once you have peeled the banana it needs to be chopped up, and it will add a thicker consistency to your smoothie if you chill or freeze it before using it. You may also want to consider chilling your strawberries. Blend until it is to the consistency you desire. Add ice cubes if you want it to thicken.

Health Benefits

Bananas aren't known to have a lot of calories, and they do help to sweeten your smoothie. This helps you to curb sugar cravings that you may be going through. Bananas are also filled with Vitamin B and Potassium. Not to mention that they boost your metabolism.

Chia seeds expand in your stomach and this helps you to feel full. This means that you will be eating less over the course of the day, which will help you to lose weight.

Iced Mocha Express

Ingredients

- 4-6 Small ice cubes
- 1 shot of expresso (brand of your choice)
- ½ cup vanilla yogurt (low fat)
- 2-3 Teaspoons Cocoa Powder (Dark is better)

Instructions

It is best to chill the expresso before using, and then add in the cocoa powder, vanilla yogurt and expresso together. Afterwards, blend on high with the Ice cubes. Add more ice cubes if you feel that you want a thicker smoothie.

Health Benefits

Cocoa powder contains some protein, so it will help you to stay fuller for longer, also, cocoa powder is a known appetite suppressant, which will help you to eat less during the day as a whole. It's also not high in calories.

Coffee Explosion

Ingredients

- 1 small banana
- ½ Teaspoon Instant coffee
- 1 Teaspoon Ginseng powder
- ½ cup chocolate soy milk
- ½ cup unsweetened almond milk

Instructions

It is usually best if you peel, chop and freeze your banana before using it. This will help to thicken your smoothie. Then blend the banana, instant coffee, and ginseng together thoroughly. Then add the soy and almond milk after pre-chilling it. Blend on high. For a thicker consistency, add ice cubes.

Health benefits

Ginseng helps to fight off fatigue and boost your energy so that you can get your day started quickly, and this helps to give you the energy you need for weight loss as well. Ginseng also helps to regulate blood sugar, which can help in weight loss as well.

Green Coffee Detoxifier

Ingredients

- 2 Teaspoons Honey (local is better)
- 1 teaspoon flax seed (ground)
- 2 Teaspoons instant Coffee
- 1 cup spinach
- ½ cup almond milk
- ½ cup low fat or 2% milk

Instructions

Mix the spinach and flax seed first, and using ground flax see is recommended. Though, to make sure that it does not turn stringy it should be blended on high. Then add the almond milk, low fat milk, honey and instant coffee. Make sure everything is chilled beforehand, as it will help to thicken your smoothie. Though, if you want your smoothie thicker you can always add ice cubes to the recipe.

Health Benefits

Honey helps to sweeten your smoothie with fewer calories than table sugar. It also has minerals and vitamins that are known to help with weight loss, as well as being known to increase your metabolism. It also helps with the digestive process which will help with weight loss over time.

Irish coffee Delight

Ingredients

- 1 teaspoon cinnamon
- ½ cup ice cubes
- 1 cup cabbage
- 1 cup chilled coffee (or 1 teaspoon of instant coffee)
- 3 tablespoons honey

Instructions

It is best to blend the cabbage first, and it won't actually be better to chill it this time. The cabbage should be prechopped and always blend on high to avoid any stringiness. Then add in the teaspoon of cinnamon, honey, and coffee. Freezing the coffee will add an extra layer of thickness. Adding in the ice cubes will then add the thickness you want to your smoothie.

Health Benefits

Cabbage is high in vitamin C which will help you to feel healthier in your day to day life while dieting. It also has lots of fiber which helps your digestive system. Cabbage is also wonderful filler that is high in various nutrients, and it doesn't add a lot of calories, making it perfect for weight loss smoothies. It also flavors easily.

Rise and Shine

Ingredients

- ½ cup fresh or frozen Mangos
- 2 teaspoons instant coffee
- ½ cup almond milk
- 1 tablespoon honey
- 1/3 cup vanilla yogurt

Instructions

The mangoes can be textured funny depending on the variety, so make sure to chop them finely and chill them before using. Freezing them is recommended. Blend them with the instant coffee, almond milk, honey, and vanilla yogurt on high until it is blended thoroughly.

Health Benefits

Using almond milk will make sure that you aren't using normal dairy, as stated before using alternative milk will make sure that your smoothies aren't too calorie rich. It will also help add more nutrients than milk can provide since it is enhanced. Using almond milk also makes your smoothies a little sweeter, and this way you won't have to use table sugar.

Berry Berry Good Coffee

Ingredients

- 1 tablespoon Flaxseed
- ½ cup blackberries
- 1 teaspoon coffee
- ½ cup low fat vanilla yogurt
- ½ cup ice cubes

Instructions

The flaxseeds are best if they are grounded, but if not you need to blend them on high. Then you can add in the blackberries, coffee, low fat vanilla yogurt and even ice cubes, of course, it will help you to thicken your smoothie if you freeze the blackberries. However, you will get more nutrients if you use fresh blackberries.

Health benefits

Flaxseed is a great way to stay full throughout the day, and it adds a bit of protein to your smoothies that would otherwise be lacking. Since it is a wonderful source of fiber it also keeps your digestive tract on the right tract, meaning you won't hold on to unnecessary weight. Some people think it gives you a boost of energy.

Good Morning Hazelnut

Ingredients

- 1 tablespoon low fat hazelnut creamer
- Frozen Iced Coffee (about six large cubes)
- ½ cup frozen raspberries
- 2/3 cup vanillas yogurt (low fat is better)

Instructions

In this recipe it is best to blend everything together, and every ingredient should be chilled if not frozen to get the proper consistency. Over blending your smoothie can weaken it and make it watery. It is best to blend on medium until the right consistency is found to avoid over blending.

Health Benefits

Raspberries are also chalk full of antioxidants that can help keep you healthy, and just like blackberries they provide a great boost of energy as well. They also have a lot of nutrients which are important when you are drinking smoothies instead of going the traditional diet route.

VEGAN SMOOTHIES

Good Morning Blueberry

Ingredients

- 1 cup Frozen Blueberries
- 1 Teaspoon honey
- ½ cup almond soy milk
- ½ banana (peeled and chopped)
- 1 teaspoon chia seeds
- 4-6 large ice cubes

Instructions

Make sure to blend the blueberries, banana, and chia seeds first. Then add in honey, soy milk and ice cubes. It is recommended to blend on high. Chilling or freezing the banana beforehand is recommended if you are looking for a thicker smoothie, but like always adding ice cubes will also thicken the smoothie.

Health Benefits

Blueberries are wonderful for weight loss, and you will find that they actually are full of vitamins and antioxidants as well. They also contain catechins, which then activate fat burning genes. You will find that blueberries are both delicious and great for you, and they add a little bit of kick to this smoothie.

The Green Lifesaver

Ingredients

- ¼ cup avocado (peeled and chopped)
- ¼ cup frozen kiwi (peeled and chopped)
- 1 green apple chopped (peeled and chopped)
- 1 tablespoon honey
- 1 teaspoon lemon juice
- 1 cup ice cubes
- ½ cup honeydew (peeled, chopped, and chilled)

Instructions

Blend the avocado, honeydew, and apple first. Then add kiwi, honey, lemon juice and ice cubes. It is best to chill or even freeze any vegetable or fruit in the smoothie. This will help your smoothie to stay at a thick consistency for longer.

Health Benefits

Green apples are rich in vitamins. Green apples are also low in calories naturally. It also has soluble fiber that will keep your body running in the right direction for weight loss, and the importance of fiber in weight loss shouldn't be forgotten.

Peach delight

Ingredients

- ½ cup Almond milk
- 1 teaspoon flaxseed oil
- 1 teaspoon honey
- ½ teaspoon ginseng powder
- 2 teaspoons chia seeds
- 1 cup frozen peaches (chopped)

Instructions

It is best to add in everything at once when it comes to this smoothie, and blend it on high to get the right consistency. Run the blender on medium if you don't want to over process your smoothie.

Health Benefits

Peaches will help to naturally sweet and best movie, and it helps you to control your calorie intake says they are excessively high. It also has many bytes will be Trans or a healthy body and help the weight loss.

Citrus Delight

Ingredients

- 1 cup soy milk
- 1 teaspoon lemon juice
- One tsp lime juice
- One orange (peeled, inspections, and chilled)
- 1 teaspoon flaxseed oil
- 6-7 ice cubes

Instructions

You can use pre-bought lime and lemon juice, but it is usually best to squeeze them fresh. Mix everything together in the blender until smooth, and then add the ice cubes until you get to the thickness of your choice. Stop adding ice cubes after you reach the desired thickness.

Health Benefits

Oranges provide a significant amount of vitamins, which helps your body to remain healthy during the weight loss process. It also keeps you regular, which will make sure you aren't keeping on unwanted weight or bloating. Better yet, oranges have very few calories, so not many calories are added to this smoothie.

Juice Power

Ingredients

- ½ cup frozen raspberries
- 1 small avocado (peeled and pitted)
- ½ cup oranges
- 2 tablespoons honey
- ½ cup frozen soy milk

Instructions

Chilling your avocado is recommended for a thicker mixture, same with your oranges. Though, it is not necessary. Just mix everything on medium until blended properly. This will usually take a few minutes since it will take time to blend the frozen fruit as well as the oranges.

Health Benefits

Raspberries are full of antioxidants and the vitamins that we need to stay healthy. When fighting against fat you need something that is high in fiber and not packed full of calories, and this is exactly what you get with raspberries, making it wonderful for weight loss smoothies.

Spinach Powerhouse

Ingredients

- 1 Cup frozen raspberries
- ½ cup fresh spinach
- ¼ cup dried oatmeal
- 12-15 ice cubes
- 8 baby carrots
- 2 teaspoons flaxseed oil

Instructions

Spinach is hard to actually blend properly, so it is best that you blend your spinach and carrots first. Having both chilled will help. Then you can add in your raspberries and oatmeal, and then you can add in your raspberries and oatmeal, and then finally your flaxseed oil and ice cubes. Only use as many ice cubes as you want to get the proper consistency that matches your tastes.

Health Benefits

Oatmeal is great for weight loss because it is high in fiber, and it will help keep you full. That's one of the reasons that oatmeal is usually used for breakfast, and staying full is extremely important when you are dealing with weight loss smoothies. Otherwise, you will end up snacking and eating more than you really should.

Almond Smoothie Delight

Ingredients

- 1 banana (sliced and frozen)
- 1 tablespoon flaxseed oil
- ½ cup almond milk
- 1 tablespoon honey
- ½ teaspoon vanilla extract

Instructions

Mix the vanilla extract, honey, flaxseed oil, and almond milk first. All of these liquids should be chilled, as it will help the consistency of your smoothie. Then add in a frozen and sliced banana. Be careful not to over blend, as it will make your smoothie weaker if you do. If so, just add more frozen banana or ice, depending upon your preference. Do not exceed one and a half bananas.

Health Benefits

Honey is going to provide you energy. Which is one of the main reasons that you are going to want honey in this smoothie? It will also give you nutrients that are needed for proper weight loss.

Cantaloupe Happiness

Ingredients

- 8-10 lettuce leaves (romaine is recommended)
- 2 cups chopped cantaloupe
- 1 cup frozen strawberries
- 5-8 ice cubes

Instructions

Lettuce leaves should be blended on high, as it will help to decrease the chances of bad texture. Then chopped, and hopefully chilled, cantaloupe, strawberries, and ice cubes can be added. Blend until the thickness desired has been reached.

Health Benefits

Cantaloupe also provides much needed fiber for weight loss, and it is low in calories while still remaining sweet. There is no abundance in sugar, but you will find some vitamins that can also help to aid in weight loss.

Tea Time is Health Time

Ingredients

- 1 cup frozen blueberries
- ½ cup acai berries
- 1 tablespoon hemp seeds
- 1 teaspoon chia seeds
- ½ Bananas
- 5-6 ice cubes
- 2 cups green tea chilled

Instructions

Make sure to blend your chia seeds and hemp seeds first, as they should be properly blended to get into your smoothie. Blend on high. Then you can add the rest of the ingredients, such as green tea, frozen blueberries, chilled acai berries, banana and ice cubes. Blend until you reach the consistency desired.

Health Benefits

Green tea is loaded with catechins, which will help your body to actually burn off fat relatively quickly. It also has some mildly energetic effects, due to the small level of caffeine it contains. Green tea is also known to help boost the metabolism.

Mango Spice Delight

Ingredients

- 1 teaspoon freshly squeezed lime juice
- ½ cup frozen mango
- 1 tablespoon flaxseed
- 2 tablespoons hemp seeds
- ¼ jalapeno
- ½ bananas
- ½ cup almond milk

Instructions

Start by blending the hemp and flaxseeds until they are to the proper consistency. Add in a little almond milk, jalapeno, mango and the lime juice. Blend until thoroughly mixed together and at the desired consistency.

Health Benefits

Mango has various nutrients, which makes it essential when limiting your calorie intake. It also helps to make sure that your smoothie is sweetened without the need for artificial sweeteners.

Tea Tree Sweet Smoothie

Ingredients

- 1 cup maple flavored tea (frozen)
- 1 frozen banana (chopped)
- ½ cup vanilla Greek yogurt
- ¼ cup chopped pecans
- 1 teaspoon cinnamon

Instructions

Make sure to blend the pecans and Greek yogurt first, and then you can add the rest of the ingredients, such as cinnamon, banana, and flavored tea. Blend until it reaches the proper consistency. You should not have pecan bits in your smoothie.

Health Benefits

Maple Flavored tea:

This all depends on the base of your tea, just avoid a black tea and this will really help. You will find that white, herbal, and other teas will provide nutrients and sometimes antioxidants that are needed for healthy weight loss.

Out of this World Cinnamon Delight

Ingredients

- ½ cup butternut squash
- ½ cup freshly squeezed orange juice (chilled)
- 2 teaspoons hemp seeds
- 1 teaspoon cinnamon
- 5-8 ice cubes

Instructions

Butternut squash should be done first, as it is harder to blend. It should be blended with hemps seeds. Then add the cinnamon, orange juice, and ice cubes. It is best to make sure that everything is chilled and precut before you put it into the blender. Blend on high for the butternut squash and hemp seeds, and then switch to medium for the rest of the ingredients.

Health Benefits

Butternut Squash is high in fiber and that is one of the main reasons that it is great for weight loss smoothies. You will find that it is also full of the much needed nutrients for weight loss smoothies, making it an excellent choice to go into the blend.

Music with a Healthy Beet

Ingredients

- ¼ cup beets (chopped)
- 2 teaspoons cinnamon
- 8-10 ice cubes
- ½ cup frozen strawberries
- ¼ cup carrots
- 1 teaspoon honey

Instructions

Even though the beets have been chopped, they should be blended first on high to avoid bad texture. Then you can add the carrots, and keep blending on high. Add frozen strawberries, cinnamon, honey and ice cubes next. Continue to blend on medium until the desired consistency has been reached.

Health Benefits

Beets are considered to be a natural weight loss food, and so they are a great addition to any weight loss smoothie. Beets are also a source of lots of fiber which can help as well. You will also find that they are full of calcium, folic acid and even iron. These are great to keep your body in balance while dieting.

Coconut Party

Ingredients

- 1 cup coconut milk
- 1 frozen banana
- ¼ cup dates
- 1 teaspoon cinnamon
- 1 cup Greek coconut yogurt
- ½ teaspoon cinnamon
- 1 cup Greek coconut yogurt
- ½ teaspoon chia seeds

Instructions

The chia seeds should be blended for about a minute on high before adding in the other ingredients. Then you can add the rest of the ingredients, such as coconut yogurt, cinnamon, dates, banana and coconut milk as blend on medium.

Health Benefits

If you grab the right type of coconut milk it is low in calories and very plenty in nutrients. Which make it perfect for a weight loss smoothie. It adds a little bit of flavor without the need for the extra calories that traditional milk can provide.

Green Bliss

Ingredients

- 1 green bell pepper
- 1 teaspoon flaxseed
- ¼ teaspoon cayenne pepper
- ¼ avocados (fresh and chilled)
- 1 green apple (chilled and in chunks)
- 10-12 ice cubes

Instructions

Everything should be chilled, and the green apple and bell pepper should be blended on high for one minute first. Then the blender can be turned on low and the avocado, cayenne pepper, flaxseed, chili powder and ice cubes can be added. Blend until it is of the right consistency. It may take about five minutes.

Health Benefit

Green Bell Peppers can aid in weight loss by providing the proper nutrients at a low calorie level, which helps you to cut out other food. It is also full of vitamins that will help to keep your body running strong.

Maca Delight

Ingredients

- 1 cup ice
- 1 teaspoon cinnamon
- 1 teaspoon maca powder
- 1 frozen banana (chopped)
- ½ Cup almond milk

Instructions

It is best to make sure that your almond milk is chilled before you use it. This will help to thicken your smoothie. Then you can blend all the ingredients together, such as cinnamon, maca powder, frozen banana, almond milk and ice. Blend on medium until smooth.

Health Benefits

Maca powder is supposed to help keep up your stamina as well as increase the chances of weight loss for that reason as well. It even can fix some hormone imbalances.

Coconut Special

Ingredients

- ½ tablespoon honey (local is recommended)
- ½ tablespoon coconut oil
- ¼ teaspoon chili powder
- ½ cup coconut milk
- ¼ cup frozen blueberries
- ½ cup medium avocado (chilled)
- 5-8 ice cubes
- 1 tablespoon spinach

Instructions

This smoothie can be blended together, and it doesn't have to be blended in stages to get the right consistency. Add in all the ingredients and blend on medium, but make sure that all the ingredients are at least chilled if you want to get the right consistency. Do not over blend, as it is easy to do with this smoothie.

Health Benefits

Honey was added to this smoothie for the nutritional value that it adds, as well as the energy that it can provide as well. Feeling fatigued is detrimental to trying to make sure that you have the energy to stick to your diet as well as the exercise regime that you've picked out for yourself, and that is what honey is supposed to help with.

Cayenne Special

Ingredients

- 2 garlic cloves
- 1 whole lime
- 1 cup avocado (chilled and chopped)
- ½ cup carrot (chilled and chopped)
- ½ cup Greek yogurt (low fat)
- 2 tablespoons honey
- ½ teaspoons honey
- ½ teaspoon cayenne pepper
- 6-8 ice cubes

Instructions

First make sure all of your ingredients are chilled, including but not limited to the garlic. Then make sure to blend your carrots and garlic on high for about one minute. Afterwards, add all other ingredients and blend on medium until you reach the desired consistency.

Health Benefits

Cayenne pepper is also known to help speed up your metabolism and curb cravings, which is why it was added.

Minty Extravaganza

Ingredients

- 2 cups spinach
- ¼ cup mint leaves
- 1 teaspoon parsley
- ¼ orange (frozen in sections)
- ¼ lime (frozen)
- ½ cucumber (chilled and chopped)
- Three small carrots
- 1 teaspoon chia seeds
- 1/3 cup Greek yogurt
- 2 tablespoons honey

Instructions

Always blend the chia seeds, mint, spinach and parsley first to make sure that it doesn't ruin the consistency of your smoothie. Blend on high for about one or two minutes, and then add the orange, lime, cucumber, carrots, Greek yogurt, and honey. Blend on medium until the consistency is right. Add ice cubes if necessary.

Health Benefits

Mint leaves have many health benefits, but they're great for weight loss as well, while adding that extra something that your smoothie needs. It's low in calories and limits the amount of sugar that is necessary to make your smoothie sweet.

Peanut Butter Perfection

Ingredients

- 2 tablespoons peanut butter
- 1 frozen banana
- 1 teaspoon cinnamon
- 1 cup Greek yogurt
- 1 tablespoon honey
- 2 teaspoons cocoa powder

Instructions

All of the ingredients can be put in together with this smoothie, and it needs to be blended on medium until it hits the right consistency. Over blending this smoothie can make it appear watery in texture.

Health Benefits

Protein is important, and it's important that you use natural protein when you are trying to lose weight as well. This is why peanut butter was added. Protein is essential when you are trying to lose weight because without it you will find that you are hungry and fatigued throughout the day. Peanut butter remedies those problems.

Vitamin Infusion

Ingredients

- 1 cup frozen papaya
- 1 tablespoon hemp seeds
- ½ cup spinach
- ½ cup green apple (frozen and chopped)
- ½ banana (frozen and chopped)
- ½ cup kale
- 5-8 ice cubes

Instructions

It is best to put the hemp seeds, spinach, and kale in first. Blend on high for about a minute or two and then add in the papaya, green apple, banana, and ice cubes. Blend on medium until it reaches the desired consistency.

Health Benefits

Hemp seeds are a great source of protein, and they help to keep you feeling a little less hungry.

Berry Berry Vitamix

Ingredients

- ¼ cup frozen blueberries
- ¼ cup strawberries (frozen and chopped)
- ¼ cup kale
- 1 cup almond milk
- 1 cup raspberries (frozen and chopped)
- ¼ cup vanilla Greek yogurt

Instructions

Blend the kale first to make sure that it isn't a weird texture. Then add in the blueberries, strawberries, almond milk, raspberries and vanilla Greek yogurt. Blend until it's the right consistency.

Health Benefits

Blueberries are full of antioxidants, which are a wonderful way to help you lose weight while still remaining healthy, and the other nutrients help as well. Blueberries also have a decent amount of fiber.

Everything is Just Peachy

Ingredients

- 1 cup almond milk
- 1 cup frozen peaches (sliced or chunks)
- 2 tablespoons flaxseed
- 1/3 cup peach Greek yogurt

Instructions

Blend the flaxseeds on high for one or two minutes. Then add in the almond milk, frozen peaches, and peach Greek yogurt. Blend on medium until you have the right consistency. Over blending can cause it to become watery in texture, In this case add ice cubes until you reach the desired consistency.

Health Benefits

Peaches were a great way to sweeten this smoothie, but you'll find that they're relatively low in calories as well. Controlling your calorie consumption is very important when you are trying to lose weight.

Chocolate Craving Smash

Ingredients

- ½ cup soy milk
- 1/3 cup vanilla Greek yogurt
- ¼ cup cocoa powder
- 1 cup fresh raspberries

Instructions

Blend everything together, but blend it on medium. You don't want to blend it on high. Otherwise, this smoothie will become too watery. You will need to make sure that you do not blend it too long.

Health Benefits

Cocoa powder actually helps you to burn the calories away while helping you remain full. It cuts off cravings as well, including sugar cravings. Not to mention that it provides that chocolate taste that is desired.

Chocolate Paradise

Ingredients

- 1 frozen banana Chopped
- 1 tablespoon chia seeds
- 2 tablespoons cocoa powder
- 1 cup almond milk
- ¼ cup vanilla extract
- 1 tablespoon raw chocolate chips
- 2 teaspoons almond butter

Instructions

First blend the chia seeds on high for about one minute. Add in the raw chocolate chips and blend on medium for about one to two minutes. Then add in the frozen banana, cocoa powder, almond milk, vanilla extract, and almond butter. Blend on medium until the desired consistency has been reached.

Health Benefits

Almond butter has a creamy texture and very few calories, making it perfect to go in a weight loss smoothie. It even has more calcium and fiber than other butters that you may use, such as peanut butter. This is also why it is healthy.

!!Bonus!!
40 + Paleo Slow Cooker Recipes

Chicken Salsa Fiesta

Ingredients

- 2 cans salsa
- 4 boneless, skinless, chicken breasts
- 1 tbsp. chili powder
- 1 onion chopped

Instructions

Coat inside of crockpot with coconut oil

Place all ingredients in a crock pot

Set the crockpot/slow cooker on low, cover and cook for 8 hours

Pull chicken apart with a fork into pieces.

Serve with gluten free tortillas, sesame crisp crackers or herb crackers. You can even serve over a salad or by itself.

Lemon Garlic Crockpot Chicken Delight

This recipe is easy to do, just place your ingredients in the crock pot and forget it, come back about 6 hours later to an awesome delicious meal.

Ingredients

- 1 whole chicken
- 30-40 cloves of garlic-peeled
- 1 whole lemon
- 1 white onion – sliced
- Salt and pepper
- Homemade Italian seasoning blend: equal parts of marjoram, thyme, rosemary, savory, sage, oregano, basil.

Instructions

Line the bottom of your pot or slow cooker with onions and garlic

Wash the chicken under cold water and pat dry

Put the chicken over the garlic and onions

Squeeze lemon juice all over the chicken

Season the inside and outside of your bird with plenty of salt, pepper and the Italian seasoning blend

Put lemon halves inside the chicken

Put the lid on the pot (or slow cooker) and let it cook on low for 6 hours, checking on it every now and again.

Place the chicken on a plate and shred the meat away off the bone.

Add meat to the broth, the garlic and onions

Discard chicken carcass.

Serve to your hungry guests.

Stuffed Peppers Galore

Ingredients

- 5 Poblano peppers or use Green peppers for a milder taste
- ½ Pound chorizo sausage browned and crumbled
- 1 Large onion – thinly sliced and browned
- 1 large tomato – diced and browned

Instructions

Cut off tops of peppers, set aside to use later

Remove seeds from inside of peppers.

Brown and crumble the sausage in a skillet

Add onions and tomatoes to skillet and cook until onions are browned.

Fill peppers with onion/sausage/tomato mixture.

Place tops on peppers to help the peppers cook faster and retain their aroma.

Coat inside of crockpot with coconut oil.

Place peppers in crockpot standing up.

Set the crockpot/slow cooker on low, cover and cook for 5-6 hours or 3-4 hours on medium.

Sione Michelson

Taste like Pizza

It's not a pizza, but if it looks like one and taste like it then why not?
Take out the cheese for a lactose free dinner.

Ingredients

Meat and sauce layer

- 1 lb. Ground beef – browned and lightly drained
- 1 cup (8 ounces) organic tomato sauce, make sure tomatoes are the only ingredient.
- 1 Tbsp. Italian seasonings
- ½ tsp garlic powder
- ½ tsp sea salt
- ½ tsp oregano

Veggie crust layer

- ½ medium, raw zucchini- grated or ground.
- 1 cup raw cauliflower – grated ground.
- 2 garlic cloves
- 2 eggs – beaten
- 3 Tbsp. coconut flour
- ¼ cup grated mozzarella cheese or cheese of choice (optional for no dairy diet)
- 1 tbsp. Butter, melted or coconut oil.
- Coconut Oil
- ¼ Tsp Sea Salt

Topping Layer

- 16 slices of pepperoni or salami
- ½ cup grated cheese of choice, I used mozzarella (optional for no dairy diet)

Instructions

Preheat oven to 400 degrees F.

Grease a large casserole dish

Brown ground beef in a large pan and drain the excess grease

Add the tomato sauce, garlic powder, Italian seasonings, sea salt and oregano.

Keep on medium heat and stir until bubbling.

Turn heat down and let it simmer for 6 minutes

In a food processor put: cauliflower, zucchini and garlic cloves.

Process it all until it resembles rice

Combine the zucchini rice, 2 eggs, ¼ cup grated cheese, ¼ tsp sea salt, 1 tbsp., melted butter and 3 tbsp. coconut flour in a different larger bowl.

Mix it all, until it resembles a kind of dough.

Coat inside of crockpot with coconut oil.

Spread ground beef evenly into the crockpot/ slow cooker

Take the vegetable dough and cover with it the top of the meat layer in the dish.

Spread it out evenly.

Place the pepperoni on the top of the crust, then sprinkle the cheese on top.

Set the crockpot/slow cooker on low, cover and cook for 3-4 hours or 2-3 hours on medium.

Brats & Sauerkraut Dinner

Ingredients

- 8 bratwurst, roughly chopped into bite-size pieces
- 1 ½ cups unpasteurized, store bought sauerkraut
- 2 green apples, peeled, cored, and chopped
- ¼ cup onion, chopped
- 1/8 cup organic honey
- 1 teaspoon caraway seeds
- 1 teaspoon red chili pepper flakes

Instructions

Place bratwurst into the slow cooker.

In a large bowl mix the sauerkraut (with the liquid), apples, onion, honey, chili, caraway seeds and pepper until well combined.

Spoon mixture into the slow cooker, over the bratwurst.

Set the slow cooker on low, cover, and cook for 5-6 hours, stirring occasionally.

Mustard & Garlic Chicken Breasts Delight

Ingredients

- 4 Chicken breasts, boneless, and skinless
- 6 tablespoons organic, unrefined coconut oil
- 4 large garlic cloves, minced
- 1 teaspoon whole grain, organic mustard
- ½ teaspoon dried oregano
- 1 ¼ teaspoon sea salt
- ½ teaspoons freshly ground black pepper
- 1 ½ teaspoons lemon zest

Instructions

In between two large sheets of wax paper pound chicken breasts until they are about ½ an inch thick with a meat mallet.

In a large zip lock bag mix together the rest of the ingredients.

Add chicken to the marinade, seal the zip lock back tightly trying to press some of the air out, and turn it several times until the chicken is well coated.

Place in a bowl and refrigerate for about 4-12 hours.

Coat inside of crockpot with coconut oil.

Place chicken breasts in crockpot, trying to keep as much of the marinade on them as possible.

Set the crockpot/slow cooker on low, cover and cook for 5-6 hours or 3-4 hours on medium.

Sione Michelson

Zesty Pork Chop Delight

Ingredients

- 4 pork chops with the bone, about ¾ inches thick each.
- 2 garlic cloves
- 1 cup fresh basil leaves, packed
- 2 tablespoons freshly squeezed lemon juice
- 1 tablespoon lemon zest
- 1 fresh chili, chopped and de-seeded (leave a few seeds in if you like hot and spicy flavors)
- 2 tablespoons extra-virgin olive oil
- 1 teaspoon coarse sea salt
- ½ teaspoons freshly ground black pepper

Instructions

With food processor running, insert garlic through the feed tube to mince.

Stop the processor and pulse the basil, and process just a couple of seconds.

Add remaining ingredients and continue to process until very well blended and thin enough to spread onto the pork chops.

Coat pork chops thoroughly with the basil mixture and marinate for 30 minutes.

Coat inside of crockpot with coconut oil.

Place pork chops in crockpot, spooning any leftover garlic herbal rub on top.

Set the crockpot/slow cooker on low, cover and cook for 5-6 hours or 3-4 hours on medium.

Allow the meat to rest a few minutes before serving.

SIDE DISH RECIPES

Wiggle Your Toes Sweet Potatoes

This recipe is my mothers and the reason why I named it "Wiggle Your Toes Sweet Potatoes" is because every time I ate them it made my toes wiggle they were so good!

Ingredients

- 2 medium sized sweet potatoes

Spice Mixture

- ½ teaspoon chili powder
- ½ teaspoon cumin
- ½ teaspoon garlic powder
- ½ teaspoon onion powder
- ½ teaspoon paprika
- ½ teaspoon sea salt
- 1/8 teaspoon ground black pepper

Sauce

- 1 tablespoon raw honey
- 2 tablespoons olive oil

Instructions

Preheat the oven to 400 degrees f.

While the oven is heating, mix together all ingredients for the spice mixture in a small bowl and set aside.

Poke small holes in the potatoes and place them all on the oven rack

Cook for 40 minutes, so the potatoes get cooked through.

Take the potatoes out of the oven, allow cooling.

Peel off skins and slice to about an inch and a half of thickness.

Place on a cookie sheet, a few inches apart.

Gently press down on each sweet potato until the sides split open slightly, which will lead to their crispiness later on.

Mix the olive oil and the honey in a bowl and drizzle half the mixture over the sweet potatoes.

Take the spice mixture and sprinkle half of the mixture over each sweet potato.

Make sure it sticks by using a spatula or your hand and pressing it.

Put the potatoes back in the oven and boil for 3-4 minutes, checking every now and then to make sure they don't burn.

Remove from oven and flip each potato over.

Drizzle the remaining sauce over the sweet potatoes, adding the remaining half of the spices.

Put back into the oven and broil for 3-4 minutes. Enjoy!

Veggie French Fries

Ingredients

- Jicama is a root veggie and is the best Paleo substitute for French fries. Jicama is also low in calories and high in nutrients.
- 1 large Jicama
- 1 tablespoon olive oil
- Sea salt and freshly ground black pepper to taste
- Paprika

Instructions

Preheat the oven to 400 F

Peel Jicama with a potato peeler.

Remove the top and bottom from the jicama and cut into French fry shapes, not too thick and not too thin.

Evenly distribute fries onto a cookie sheet, being careful not to overlap.

Sprinkle with olive oil

Sprinkle with sea seasonings

Bake for about 20 minutes, or until desired doneness. We all like our fries a little bit different from just a little bit crunchy to super crunchy.

Sione Michelson

Cauliflower Rice Delight

Ingredients

- 1 head of cauliflower
- 4 tablespoons lard
- 4 carrots – peeled and chopped
- 1 small onion – chopped
- 2 tablespoons garlic – chopped
- 1 cup green peas
- 4 eggs – whisked
- 6 tablespoons coconut aminos
- ½ teaspoon sesame oil
- ½ teaspoon fish sauce
- Sea salt and ground pepper to taste

Instructions

Whisk the eggs

Place cauliflower in food processor and pulse until it resembles the size of rice.

Heat your skillet or wok over medium to high heat.

Add 2 tablespoons of lard to the pan and let it melt.

Add the garlic, onions and carrots and cook for 3 minutes.

Add peas and cook for one more minute. Remove from pan and set aside.

In a separate pan, add your whisked eggs and scramble them, so they gain a slightly brown color. Add the salt and pepper.

Place vegetables in a large bowl.

Add 2 tablespoons of fat to the pan allow melting.

Add the cauliflower rice to the pan coating with the oil. Cook for about 5-7 minutes, stirring every now and then until crispy

Add the reserved vegetables back in the pan and stir well.

Next add the coconut aminos, sesame oil, fish sauce. Add pepper and salt to taste.

Serve and enjoy!

Ginger Carrots with an Orange Twist

You like carrots with your steak than this dish is a nice complement to a juicy steak.

Ingredients

- 1 pound carrots – peeled and cut into ½" slices
- 1 cup water
- Dash sea salt
- 1 tablespoon lard or bacon fat
- 1 orange – save both the juice and zest
- 2 tablespoons raw honey
- ½ teaspoon ground ginger
- Ground black pepper

Instructions

Place the salt and the water in a saucepan.

Add the carrots and bring the water to a boil.

Next, reduce the heat and let simmer for 5 minutes until carrots are soft

Drain the water.

Add the remaining ingredients (orange, Honey and ginger) to the pan.

Stir to combine and sauté for 2-3 minutes until carrots are very soft and the glaze is slightly thicker.

Add salt and pepper to taste.

The Best Mushroom Side dish

Ingredients

- 1 pound mushrooms
- 2-3 tablespoons olive oil
- 1 tablespoon balsamic vinegar
- 3-5 cloves garlic – minced or pressed
- 3 pinches dried thyme
- 1.2 pinches cayenne pepper
- ¼ teaspoon freshly freshly cracked pepper
- 1-2 tablespoons fresh parsley, chopped

Instructions

Preheat oven to 400 degrees F.

Wipe the mushroom clean.

Leave them whole and only cut them if they are large.

Combine the olive oil, balsamic vinegar, thyme, cayenne, garlic, salt and pepper in a bowl and mix.

Coat the mushrooms with this mixture.

Place mushrooms on a large baking sheet.

Roast in oven for 20-30 minutes

Serve with fresh parsley.

Sione Michelson

Spicy Tuna Salad Delight

Ingredients

- 2 cans tuna, water packed, drained
- 20 (About 1 Cup) Green or black olives – chopped
- 2 green onions- chopped
- 1 jalapeno pepper – finely chopped
- 3 tbsp. capers – rinsed
- ½ Tsp red chili flakes
- Juice of 2 lemons
- Splash of olive oil
- 1 head butter lettuce, kale or mixed greens
- 1 avocado – sliced

Instructions

Combine the first 8 ingredients, mix well.

Serve over greens.

Place sliced avocado on top. Serve with gluten free tortillas, sesame crisp crackers or herb crackers.

Pomegranate Salad Delight

Ingredients

- 1 head escarole or Arugula lettuce, washed, dried, and torn into bite sized pieces
- 1 pomegranate, seeds removed.
- 5 tablespoons extra virgin olive oil
- 2 garlic cloves, minced
- 2 tablespoons freshly ground black pepper to taste

Instructions

In a jam type jar combine oil, lemon juice, garlic, salt, pepper, and shake.

In a large serving bowl combine the lettuce and pomegranate seeds and with clean hands mix well to blend the seeds into the salad.

Shake the dressing again and toss into the salad and serve.

Sione Michelson

Arugula Avocado and Raisins Salad

Ingredients

- Two large handfuls arugula leaves, washed and dried well
- 1 avocado, cut in half, seeded, and sliced thinly
- ½ cup organic raisins
- ½ thinly sliced Spanish onion (red onion)
- 6 cherry tomatoes, sliced in half lengthwise
- 6 tablespoons extra virgin olive oil
- 2 tablespoons freshly squeezed lemon juice
- Sea salt and freshly ground black pepper to taste

Instructions

In a jar mix the dressing ingredients along with the salt and pepper and shake.

In a large bowl, gently mix together the salad ingredients.

Shake the dressing a second time and dress the salad with it.

Serve immediately

Apple Coleslaw Delight

Ingredients

- Very finely sliced white cabbage, about 2 cups
- 2 medium sized carrots, shredded
- 1 apple, chopped
- 1 stalk of celery, chopped
- 1 green onion, sliced thinly, discard the dark green part
- 1 handful toasted sunflower seeds
- ¼ cup extra virgin olive oil
- 2 tablespoons organic honey
- 1 tablespoon freshly squeezed lemon juice
- Sea salt and freshly ground black pepper to taste

Instructions

In a jar shake together the liquid ingredients and the salt and pepper to blend.

Let it sit while you prepare the coleslaw so the salt dissolves. Taste it to see if it needs a little more of anything.

In a large bowl mix together the veggies.

Shake the dressing ingredients one last time and pour over the coleslaw and toss well.

Sprinkle the sunflower seeds over the top and toss again.

Let sit for about 15 minutes and serve.

Mediterranean Salad

Ingredients

- Juice of ½ to 1 lemon (depending upon how lemon-y you like it)
- 3 Tbsp. olive oil
- 1 clove garlic, minced
- ¼ Tsp red pepper flakes
- ½ Tsp dried oregano
- ¼ tsp sea salt
- Freshly ground black pepper
- 1 bunch lacinato kale – with no stems and well washed

Topping:

- ¼-1/2 LB. Hard Salami, diced
- ½ cup pickled sweet peppers or cherry tomatoes
- ½ cup pepperoncini
- 4-6 marinated artichoke hearts
- ¼ cup green olives
- ¼ cup toasted sunflower seeds
- 4-6 pickled red onion slices or rings (optional)
- Roasted cauliflower (optional)

Instructions

In a jar with a lid, combine lemon juice, olive oil, garlic, oregano, red pepper flakes, pepper and salt.

Close with the lid and blend it by shaking vigorously.

Slice kale leaves thinly and toss them in a bowl.

Coat kale with the lemon dressing.

Combine the remaining 8 ingredients to create topping.

Place kale in individual salad bowls.

Sprinkle topping over the kale.

APPETIZER RECIPES

Sesame Crunch Crackers

Ingredients

- ½ cup dates
- ½ cup raisins
- ¼ cup each of sunflower seeds, pepitas, and sesame seeds
- ¼ cup each of almond flour and flaxseed meal
- ½ teaspoon sea salt
- 2 tablespoons water

Instructions

Preheat oven to 275 degrees F

Pulse dates and raisins together in food processor. Grind evenly.

Add in all the seeds, almonds, salt, flour, meal and the water.

Blend together well until it is sticking together.

Roll the dough between two parchment papers until they get really thin (approximately 1/8 inch thickness). Do this in 2 or 3 batches. Bake for 30 minutes, until lightly browned, nice and crispy. Use a sharp knife to cut them into equal size chips. Let cool.

Herbs Galore Crackers

Ingredients

- 2 cups Almond flour
- ½ teaspoon sea salt
- 2 tablespoons your favorite herbs of choice, with rosemary
- 2 tablespoons water
- 1 egg white
- 1 tablespoon olive oil
- ¼ teaspoon coconut oil

Instructions

Preheat oven to 350 degrees F.

Combine salt, almond flour and herbs in a medium bowl.

Combine the egg white, olive oil, water, and melted coconut oil. Whisk ingredients together.

Add the wet ingredients to the flour ingredients in first bowl and stir until a dough forms.

Add water or oil only if it doesn't stick together as a dough ball.

Place dough between two sheets of parchment paper. Roll out to an even thickness of ¼ inch thick.

Transfer parchment to a baking sheet pan and remove the top parchment. Trim the edges and cut the dough into crackers.

Bake for 10 minutes; let them set in the oven for 10 minutes with the heat turned off.

Rolls de Sweet Potato

Ingredients

- ½ cup cooked yam or sweet potato
- ¼ cup blanched almond flour
- 1 ½ cups tapioca flour
- 1 teaspoon baking powder
- 1 teaspoon sea salt
- ¼ cup almond milk
- ¼ cup olive oil
- 1 large egg
- 1 tablespoon ghee (optional)

Instructions

Heat oven to 400 degrees F.

Combine the almond flour with the tapioca flour, the baking powder and the sea salt in a bowl. Mix on low speed, with a mixer, until well blended.

Do this; slowly add half of the flour mixture from the first bowl.

Mix the dough with your hands adding the remaining half the flour until gone. Knead for 2 minutes until it stops being sticky. Cover the dough with a kitchen towel and set aside for 10 minutes.

Roll the dough out into equal balls and place on a baking sheet covered with parchment paper, making sure there is enough space between each ball. Bake in the oven for 14-17 minutes and the tops get light brown.

Allow to cool for 15-20 minutes.

Sione Michelson

Apple Cinnamon Treats

Ingredients

- 1-2 apples
- 1 Tsp. Cinnamon

Instructions

Preheat oven to 200 degrees F

Slice the apple into very thin slices and take out the seeds.

Line the slices on a baking sheet covered in parchment paper.

Leave space between the slices.

Sprinkle with cinnamon.

Bake the slices for 1 hour, and then flip them over.

Continue baking and flipping for 1-2 hours, until they're dry throughout.

Tortillas Paleo Style

Ingredients

- 1 cup blanched almond flour
- 1 cup tapioca flour
- ½ Tsp. seal salt
- 4 Tbsp. light olive oil
- 6 tbsp. warm water

Instructions

Dip the measuring cup into the almond flour and scrape the top, to make sure you get exactly 1 cup.

Whisk together the almond flour, tapioca and sea salt

Add oil to the flour mixture and stir until the flour is blended thoroughly.

Add the water to the bowl and stir until well combined.

On a flat surface, knead the dough for 1 minute.

Cut the dough into 8 pieces and knead each well for about 30 seconds.

Roll each piece into a ball between two pieces of parchment paper

Flatten with a tortilla press or rolling pin

Place the tortilla into a heated skillet and cook for 30 seconds to 1 minute

Flip over and cook for another 30 seconds to 1 minute

Use with any recipe calling for tortillas.

Sione Michelson

DESSERT RECIPES

Gluten Free Brownies

Ingredients

- ½ cup ghee
- ½ cup maple syrup
- 3 ½ ounces dark chocolate that is 85% cocoa
- 5 organic free range eggs
- 1/3 cup coconut flour
- ¼ cup powdered cocoa
- ¼ teaspoon Paleo friendly baking powder
- ½ teaspoon baking soda
- ½ teaspoon real vanilla extract.

Instructions

In a large bowl, mix together all the dry ingredients.

In an electric mixing bowl beat together the eggs and maple syrup until completed mixed

Now add the dry ingredients and beat again until all ingredients are well combined.

Melt chocolate and butter in a double boiler pan

Add the melted chocolate to the above mixture and blend it by hand until it has a thick consistency.

Place the batter in a small square baking pan, oiled and floured, of about 8 ½ inches wide.

Bake at 350 degrees Fahrenheit for 20 to 25 minutes or until a toothpick inserted in the middle comes out clean.

Allow to cool before removing from pan.

Banana Bread Delight

Ingredients

- ½ cup coconut flour
- ¾ cup almond flour
- ½ teaspoon powdered cinnamon
- 1 teaspoon baking soda
- 3 tablespoons organic honey
- 4 organic free range eggs, separate the whites from the yolks in separate bowls
- ½ teaspoon vanilla extract
- 1 ½ cup bananas, puree
- ¼ cup cocoa grains
- 2 tablespoons coconut milk

Instructions

Heat oven to 375 degrees F.

Mix together all the dry ingredients in a large mixing bowl.

In another large mixing bowl mix together the egg yolks, vanilla extract, and honey.

Add the banana puree and mix again.

Add the dry ingredients and cocoa grains, mix well.

Beat the egg whites until they are frothy and thick.

If the mixture feels too thick, add a little more coconut milk.

Oil and flour an 8 inch by 4 inch baking pan.

Bake for 45 minutes, or until you stick a toothpick inside and it comes out dry. Cool bread for about 20 minutes.

Sione Michelson

German Carrot Cake Delight

Ingredients

- 6 eggs- separated
- ½ cup raw honey (less, if desired)
- 1 ½ cup cooked and pureed carrots
- 1 Tbsp. Orange Zest
- 1 Tbsp. Orange juice (freshly squeezed)
- 3 cups almond flour
- Coconut oil

Instructions

Preheat oven to 325 degrees F.

Whisk together the honey and egg yolks.

Add orange zest and juice, almond flour and carrot puree.

Whisk the egg whites in a separate bowl until they stiffen, then fold into batter.

Pour batter into a coconut oil greased pan.

Bake for 50 minutes, when a skewer piercing through the center of the cake comes out clean.

Cool in the pan for 15 minutes, then take it out and let it cool.

Blueberry Brownies Delight

Ingredients

- 1 cup coconut cream concentrate – melted
- 3 eggs
- ½ cup raw organic honey
- 1 cup blueberries
- 1 cup pecans – crushed
- ¼ cup organic cocoa powder
- 1 Tbsp. Cinnamon
- 1 Tbsp. ground coffee of your choice
- 2 tsp vanilla extract
- ½ Tsp baking soda
- ¼ Tsp sea salt

Instructions

Preheat oven to 325 degrees F

Place all the ingredients in a mixing bowl except blueberries.

Use a mixer to blend them well

Add the blueberries by hand.

Pour your batter into a greased baking dish

Bake for 30 minutes. Test it after 25 minutes.

Once cool, use melted coconut cream concentrate, to drizzle over brownies.

Cut, serve, and enjoy!

The Best Dessert Tapioca Crepes

Ingredients

- 1 cup tapioca flour or starch
- 1 cup full fat canned coconut milk
- 1 egg
- Pinch sea salt
- Toppings of choice (see suggestions below)

Instructions

Combine all the ingredients and mix until it's all smooth.

Pour in a hot pan about 1/3 cup of mixture and spread it out, by tilting the pan. These will be a lot thinner than pancakes.

Cook both sides until they become slightly brown. Check them often.

For breakfast, serve with maple syrup or honey and bacon or sausages.

Sweet Apple Feast

Ingredients

- 6 Apples- peeled, cored and sliced
- 1 Cup water
- 2 Tbsp. Fresh Lemon Juice
- 2 Tbsp. chopped dried cherries (unsweetened)
- ½ cup chopped dried apricots
- 2 Tsp. ground cinnamon
- ¼ Tsp ground ginger
- ¼ Tsp ground cloves
- ¼ Tsp ground nutmeg
- 2 Tbsp. ghee (clarified butter)
- 1 Tbsp. fresh lemon zest.

Instructions

Combine the water with the apples and lemon juice in a large saucepan

Bring them to a boil.

Cover the pan and let it simmer for 25 minutes, until apples are tender.

Add in the apricots, dried cherries, ginger, cinnamon, cloves and nutmeg.

Stir and cook for 5 minutes.

Add ghee to the mix and stir until melted.

Add lemon zest.

BREAKFAST

Chorizo Sausage & eggs

Prep time: 20 minutes

Cooking Time: 9 hours

Ingredients

- 1 lb. chorizo sausage
- 1 small onion
- 12 eggs
- 1 cup coconut milk
- 1 small butternut squash
- Ghee/ oil for greasing the crockpot

Instructions

Place the chorizo in a skillet, and let it cook.

Cut up the onions.

Add the onion to the skillet, cooking just until the onion is soft. You don't need to finish cooking the sausage; it will finish in the crockpot preventing sticking.

Add your squash, the sausage/ onion mixture and then the egg/ milk mixture.

Turn crockpot on low for 8-10 hours. Wake up, eat and enjoy!

Sweet Breakfast Carnitas

Prep Time: 30 Minutes

Cook time: 8 hours

Ingredients

- 1 Tsp cinnamon
- 1 Tsp dried parsley
- ½ Tsp. dried sage
- ¼ Tsp nutmeg
- Salt and pepper, to taste
- 4 to 5 strips of bacon
- 2 cups blueberries
- ¼ cup of maple syrup
- Fresh parsley chopped (to garnish)
- 2 to 3 lb. Pork shoulder roast
- ½ cup apple juice

Instructions

Set the roast inside the slow cooker and pour the apple juice in, followed by the maple syrup.

Sprinkle the nutmeg, salt and pepper, dried sage, cinnamon, and dried parsley on top of the roast. Gently pat with fingers to make sure it stays.

Add a few raspberries to serve as a topping.

Cook on low setting for 8 hours

Remove the meat from the cooker and set it aside. Shred the meat.

To help keep the meat moist, add the remaining liquids to the meat.

Cook the bacon on the stove top and place on paper towels to drain excess grease.

Once the bacon is cool, crumble it into tiny pieces and add at least half to the shredded pork.

Warm your bacon fat pan on medium-high heat and with the help of a large spoon, collect both the bacon and pork. Using your hands press down flat in the skillet and cook each side for about 3 minutes, until they are nice and crispy. Serve hot.

Slow Cooker Casserole Paleo Style

Prep Time: 10 minutes

Cooking Time: 6 hours

Ingredients

- 2 teaspoons of minced garlic
- 1 cup of kale (roughly chopped)
- 2 tablespoons of coconut oil
- 1.5 cups of sliced leeks
- 1.5 cups of shredded sweet potato
- 1.5 cups of beef sausage
- 8 large eggs beaten

Instructions

Melt coconut oil over medium heat in a pan.

Add the kale, garlic and leeks and sauté.

Add the sweet potato, beef sausage, eggs and sautéed vegetables to your slow cooker, and cook it on low for 6 hours.

Let it cool down completely.

Divide into equally cut pieces and freeze in freezer bags.

Heat in the microwave for about 2 minutes, and then serve.

Pumpkin Stew Delight

Prep Time: 20 minutes

Cooking time: 7 to 8 hours

Ingredients

- 2 lbs. of grass fed stew meat, cubed
- 4 cups of butternut squash, cubed
- 1 medium onion, chopped
- 1 cup of dried cherries
- 2 teaspoons of sage
- 1 tablespoon of thyme
- 1 bay leaf
- 4 cups of beef stock
- 1 teaspoon of allspice
- ½ teaspoon of nutmeg
- 1 cup of pumpkin, pureed
- 1 teaspoon of salt
- 1 teaspoon of ground black pepper

Instructions

In a saucepan, heat the coconut oil and sauté the chopped onions, sage, thyme on medium heat until the onions look translucent.

In a high heat skillet, sear the meat until a brown crust forms.

Pour the onion mixture and the meat into the crock-pot. Add the beef stock, nutmeg, bay leaf, and allspice. Put this on low heat for 6 hours.

After 6 hours, add the cubed butternut squash and dried cherries. Set on low heat for another 1-2 hours.

Before serving, add pureed pumpkin as desired. Then season with salt and pepper and other spices, if you would like to.

Crockpot Breakfast Delight

Prep Time: 10 minutes

Cooking time: 8 hours

Ingredients

- 2 pounds of ground beef
- 8 eggs, whisked
- 2 pieces of sweet potato, shredded
- 1 sweet onion, diced
- 1 tablespoon of garlic powder
- 2 teaspoons dried basil
- 1 teaspoon salt
- 1 teaspoon black pepper
- Any vegetable you want to add (Squash, chayote, etc.)

Instructions

Add all the ingredients: (whisked eggs, shredded sweet potato, ground beef, diced sweet onion, garlic powder, dried basil, seasonings, and extra vegetables you might want to include) to your slow cooker and mix well using a ladle.

Place on low temperature for 6 to 8 hours.

Take it out and let it cool for 5 minutes.

Serve and enjoy!

Sweet Eggs

Prep Time: 5 minutes

Cooking time: 4.5 hours

Ingredients

- 1 dozen eggs
- 2-4 teabags
- 6-8 cups of water
- 2 tablespoons of cinnamon
- 1 teaspoon of ground black pepper
- 1 teaspoon of salt

Instructions

Place the eggs in a pot filled with water and put on low heat for about 30 minutes or until hard boiled.

After the eggs are hard boiled, take them out and place them in a bowl of cold water.

Crack the shell of the eggs but do not peel them.

Place the cracked eggs in the pot filled with 6-8 cups of water.

Leave the teabags inside the pot with the strings out and cover the pot with the lid.

Let this simmer for about 30 minutes

Remove the teabags and let the eggs simmer for about 3.5 hours with the lid on.

Take the eggs from the pot and let them cool. Peel off the shell and place the unshelled eggs in a bowl. Sprinkle salt, black pepper, and cinnamon over them. Serve!

You can use a slow cooker for this if desired. Simply leave tea bags with eggs for 2 hours and continue cooking on high heat for 6 more hours. In a slow cooker it will take 8 hours total time.

Closing

Again I want to thank you for checking out my book and I hope you enjoyed these delicious & healthy juice recipes. You now have one weapon in your arsenal (this e-book) that will surely help you towards the battle against fat and obesity by cutting out the main culprit of your weight gain which is un-wanted carbs. As you take your Juicing Cleanse Journey hopefully beyond this book is sure you take action every day and Never GIVE UP!

I urge you to continue to add new weapons in your arsenal and if you have setbacks just keep going because all the hard work you put in will definitely be well worth it. I wish you a prosperous and healthy life, BE WELL SPIRITUALLY, PHYSICALLY AND EMOTIONALLY!

Get All My Books to Help in Mastering your Life Today

JUICING: THE ULTIMATE BEGINNERS GUIDE FOR JUICING WITH THE NINJA BLENDER & NUTRIBULLET (OVER 60 RECIPES NEW!!!!)) (Juicing, Juicing for Weight Loss, Books, Recipes, ... for Weight Loss, Women's Health Diet)

Paleo Diet:: Learn How to Lose Weight and Feel Amazing in just 5 Short Weeks. The Quickest way to Fit into that Swimsuit for Summer! (Paleo Made Easy) (Paleo ... Diet, Slow Cooker, Recipes, Diet Recipes)

Paleo Diet: Why The Paleo Diet is better for you than the Low Fat High Carb Diet & the Paleo Recipes that will help Save Your Life! (Paleo Cookbook, Weight-Loss, ... Diet, Slow Cooker, Recipes, Diet Recipes)

Paleo Diet: 7 Days To Better Health: Cure Your Acid Reflux, Heartburn, Start losing Weight, Lower Blood Pressure and Cholesterol All in a Week through ... Diet, Slow Cooker, Recipes, Diet Recipes)

Juicing: The Ultimate 7 Day Juicing Cleanse for Weight-loss Guide: Over 60 Delicious Juicing Recipes made with the Nutribullet and Ninja. Increase Metabolism ... Weight Loss, Women's Health Diet Book 1)

Juicing: The Ultimate 7 Day Juice Challenge: (60+recipes!!) To help Lower your Blood Pressure, Cholesterol, Acid Reflux and Start Losing Weight all with ... Weight Loss, Women's Health Diet Book 1)

The Low Carb Nutribullet & Ninja Recipe Book: 10 day juice cleanse: 100+ Health Sustaining Low Carb and Delicious and Nutritious Juice and Smoothie Recipes ... for Weight Loss, Women's Health Diet)

Juicing: The Only Juicing for Health Guide You Will Ever Need:100 + Juicing and Smoothie Recipes for Weight Loss, Lower Blood Pressure, Reduce Acid Reflux ... for Weight Loss, Women's Health Diet)

Juicing for Health: The Ultimate Juicing Guide for Optimal Health: Start Feeling Better your Very First Day: 100+ Easy To Follow Nutribullet & Ninja Recipes. ... for Weight Loss, Women's Health Diet)

Juicing for Fat Loss: The Ultimate Juicing Guide for Fat Loss: A complete 10 Day Juicing Guide that is Sure to Help You Lose Fat and Keep it off for Good!

Juicing For Beginners: The Easiest Juicing Guide Ever Made, 100+ Delicious Juicing and Smoothie Recipes for Optimal Health, Lower your Blood Pressure & ... for Weight Loss, Women's Health Diet)

Juicing: Juicing for Vitality: 7 Days to a Better Life, Drastically Improve your Energy, Lose Weight, Improve Sex Drive, Improve Skin Complexion and Much ... for Weight Loss, Women's Health Diet)

Juicing: Juicing for Weight Loss: 5 Days to Better Health, Easy to Follow Steps and Recipes: Lose Weight & Improve Your Health all by Taking Action Today! ... for Weight Loss, Women's Health Diet)

www.ingramcontent.com/pod-product-compliance
Lightning Source LLC
Chambersburg PA
CBHW070423290526
45791CB00005B/1807